ADVANCES IN

Vascular Surgery

VOLUME 9

ADVANCES IN

Vascular Surgery

VOLUMES 1 THROUGH 5 (OUT OF PRINT)

ADVANCES IN

Vascular Surgery

VOLUME 9

Editor-in-Chief
Anthony D. Whittemore, MD
Chief Medical Officer, Chief, Division of Vascular Surgery, Brigham and Women's Hospital; Professor of Surgery, Harvard Medical School, Boston, Massachusetts

Associate Editors
Dennis F. Bandyk, MD
Professor of Surgery; Director, Vascular Surgery Division, University of South Florida College of Medicine, Tampa

Jack L. Cronenwett, MD
Professor of Surgery, Dartmouth Medical School; Chief, Section of Vascular Surgery, Dartmouth–Hitchcock Medical Center, Lebanon, New Hampshire

Norman R. Hertzer, MD
Department of Vascular Surgery, Cleveland Clinic Foundation, Cleveland, Ohio

Rodney A. White, MD
Professor of Surgery, University of California at Los Angeles School of Medicine; Chief of Vascular Surgery, Associate Chairman, Department of Surgery, Harbor–University of California at Los Angeles Medical Center, Torrance

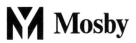 Mosby

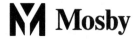 Mosby

Publisher: Cynthia Baudendistel
Developmental Editor: Karen Moehlman
Manager, Continuity Production: Idelle L. Winer
Production Editor: Donna Skelton
Project Supervisor, Production: Joy Moore
Composition Specialist, Production: Betty Dockins

Printed in the United States of America
Printing/binding by The Maple-Vail Book Manufacturing Group

Editorial Office:
Mosby, Inc.
11830 Westline Industrial Drive
St. Louis, MO 63146
Customer Service: hhspcs@harcourt.com

International Standard Serial Number: 1069-7292
International Standard Book Number: 0-8151-2731-6

Contributors

Sonia S. Anand, MD, MSc
Assistant Professor of Medicine, Department of Medicine, McMaster University, and Vascular Medicine Specialist, Hamilton Health Sciences Corporation, Hamilton, Ontario, Canada

P.R.F. Bell, MB, ChB, MD, FRCS
Professor of Surgery, University of Leicester, Leicester Royal Infirmary, Leicester, England

John J. Bergan, MD, FACS, FRCS (Hon) Eng
Clinical Professor of Surgery, University of California, San Diego; Clinical Professor of Surgery, Uniformed Services University of the Health Sciences, Bethesda, Md

Bruce J. Brener, MD
Associate Clinical Professor of Surgery, Columbia University, and Chief, Vascular Surgery, Newark Beth Israel Medical Center, Newark, NJ

Ruth L. Bush, MD
Vascular Surgery Fellow, Division of Vascular Surgery, Emory University School of Medicine, Atlanta, Ga

Elliot L. Chaikof, MD, PhD
Associate Professor of Surgery, Division of Vascular Surgery, Emory University School of Medicine, Atlanta, Ga

Daniel G. Clair, MD
Vice Chairman, Vascular Surgery, Cleveland Clinic Foundation, Cleveland, Ohio

Richard D. Fessler, MD
Associate Clinical Professor of Neurological Surgery, Wayne State University, Director of Neuroendovascular Surgery, Harper University Hospital–Detroit Medical Center, Detroit, Michigan

Robert A. Fitridge, MS, FRACS
Senior Lecturer in Vascular Surgery, University of Adelaide, and Consultant Vascular Surgeon and Head of Vascular Unit, The Queen Elizabeth Hospital, Adelaide, Australia

Samuel Z. Goldhaber, MD
Associate Professor of Medicine, Harvard Medical School, and Director, Venous Thromboembolism Research Group, Brigham and Women's Hospital, Boston, Mass

Lee R. Guterman, PhD, MD
Assistant Professor of Neurosurgery, Department of Neurosurgery and Toshiba Stroke Research Center, School of Medicine and Biomedical Sciences, University at Buffalo, State University of New York, Buffalo

Jennifer A. Heller, MD
Clinical Fellow, Division of Vascular Surgery, New York Presbyterian Hospital, Cornell Campus, New York, NY

L. Nelson Hopkins, MD
Professor and Chairman of Neurosurgery, Department of Neurosurgery and Toshiba Stroke Research Center, School of Medicine and Biomedical Sciences, University at Buffalo, State University of New York, Buffalo

K. Craig Kent, MD
Professor of Surgery, Weill Medical College of Cornell University, Chief, Division of Vascular Surgery, Director, Vascular Center, New York Presbyterian Hospital, New York, NY

Lee Kirksey, MD
Fellow in Vascular Surgery, Newark Beth Israel Medical Center, St. Barnabas Health Care System, Newark, NJ

Giuseppe Lanzino, MD
Chief Resident, Department of Neurosurgery, University of Virginia Health Sciences Center, Charlottesville

Peter H. Lin, MD
Assistant Professor of Surgery, Division of Vascular Surgery, Emory University School of Medicine, Atlanta, Ga

Alan B. Lumsden, MD
Associate Professor of Surgery, Chief, Division of Vascular Surgery, Emory University School of Medicine, Atlanta, Ga

John H. Matsuura, MD
Assistant Professor of Surgery, Medical College of Georgia, Augusta, Atlanta Medical Center, Atlanta, Ga

Takao Ohki, MD
Associate Professor of Surgery, Albert Einstein College of Medicine, and Chief, Endovascular Program, Montefiore Medical Center, New York, NY

Don Poldermans, MD, PhD, FESC
Consultant, Internal Medicine, Department of Vascular Surgery, Erasmus Medical Centre, Rotterdam, The Netherlands

Adnan I. Qureshi, MD
Assistant Professor of Neurosurgery, Department of Neurosurgery and Toshiba Stroke Research Center, School of Medicine and Biomedical Sciences, University at Buffalo, State University of New York, Buffalo

Andrew J. Ringer, MD
Assistant Professor of Clinical Neurosurgery, University of Cincinnati, Cincinnati, Ohio

David Rosenthal, MD
Clinical Professor of Surgery, Medical College of Georgia, Augusta, Chief of Vascular Surgery, Atlanta Medical Center, Atlanta, Ga

Hero van Urk, MD, PhD
Professor Vascular Surgery, Head and Department of Vascular Surgery, Erasmus Medical Centre, Rotterdam, The Netherlands

Frank J. Veith, MD
Professor of Surgery, Albert Einstein College of Medicine, and Chief, Vascular Surgery, Montefiore Medical Center, New York, NY

Victor J. Weiss, MD
Assistant Professor of Surgery, Division of Vascular Surgery, Emory University School of Medicine, Atlanta, Ga

Rodney A. White, MD
Professor of Surgery, University of California at Los Angeles School of Medicine; Chief, Vascular Surgery, Associate Chairman, Department of Surgery, Harbor-UCLA Medical Center, Torrance, Calif

Contents

PART I

Carotid Artery Disease

CHAPTER 1

Carotid Angioplasty and Stenting: The Neurosurgical Perspective

Andrew J. Ringer, MD
Assistant Professor of Clinical Neurosurgery, University of Cincinnati, Cincinnati, Ohio

Giuseppe Lanzino, MD
Chief Resident, Department of Neurosurgery, University of Virginia Health Sciences Center, Charlottesville

Richard D. Fessler, MD
Associate Clinical Professor of Neurological Surgery, Wayne State University, Director of Neuroendovascular Surgery, Harper University Hospital–Detroit Medical Center, Detroit, Michigan

Adnan I. Qureshi, MD
Assistant Professor of Neurosurgery, Department of Neurosurgery and Toshiba Stroke Research Center, School of Medicine and Biomedical Sciences, University at Buffalo, State University of New York, Buffalo

Lee R. Guterman, PhD, MD
Assistant Professor of Neurosurgery, Department of Neurosurgery and Toshiba Stroke Research Center, School of Medicine and Biomedical Sciences, University at Buffalo, State University of New York, Buffalo

L. Nelson Hopkins, MD
Professor and Chairman of Neurosurgery, Department of Neurosurgery and Toshiba Stroke Research Center, School of Medicine and Biomedical Sciences, University at Buffalo, State University of New York, Buffalo

Carotid endarterectomy (CEA) is now widely accepted as the standard of care for significant symptomatic or asymptomatic carotid artery stenosis. The ability of CEA to improve outcome depends in large part on the morbidity of the procedure, sparking a debate regarding the management of certain "high-risk" patients. In addition, patient preference has driven a trend toward less-invasive methods of treatment for a wide variety of disorders, and carotid stenosis has been no exception. As a result, carotid angioplasty and stenting (CAS) is gaining popularity as an alternative to CEA for high-risk patients with severe carotid stenosis and may be considered as an alternative to open surgery for patients who desire a less-invasive therapy. The wisdom of this alternative will depend on the safety and efficacy of CAS relative to CEA and is discussed in this chapter. The mechanism of CAS, criteria for patient selection, perioperative management, operative technique, and methods of complication avoidance are reviewed.

MECHANISM OF ACTION

Unlike CEA, in which the aim is to remove the offending pathology, the mechanism of carotid angioplasty is much different. Angioplasty within a stenotic lesion results in fracture of the plaque and stretching of the media.[1] The result is often a normal or near-normal lumen size with new irregularities within the plaque that may serve as thrombogenic sites before remodeling and endothelialization occur.[2,3] As a result, perioperative management with antiplatelet agents is paramount. In addition, the risk of embolization is high during fracture of the plaque. The clinical correlate to this risk is the relatively high incidence of perioperative transient ischemic attacks (TIAs) after CAS, relative to CEA. In an attempt to minimize this risk, intraoperative distal protection techniques have been described and are currently under development. The use of these techniques as well as the perioperative regimen for prophylaxis against embolism will be discussed in detail later in this chapter.

CHOOSING THE APPROPRIATE PATIENT

Several large cooperative randomized trials have proved the efficacy of CEA for extracranial carotid artery stenosis.[4-6] The rigid selection criteria used by these trials, however, makes the application of their results to everyday practice difficult. In the North American Symptomatic Carotid Endarterectomy Trial (NASCET),[6] European Carotid Surgery Trial,[4] and Asymptomatic Carotid Atherosclerosis Study (ACAS),[5] the investigators sought to eliminate any factors that might complicate the interpretation of treatment outcomes. These factors included age older than 79 years; heart, kidney, liver, or lung failure; cancer likely to cause death within 5 years; cardiac valvular lesion or rhythm disorder likely to be associated with cardioembolic stroke; previous ipsilateral CEA; angina or myocardial infarction in the previous 6 months; progressing neurologic signs; contralateral CEA within 4 months; or a major surgical procedure within 30 days. The result is that a large number of patients with significant carotid artery disease were not included in these studies, and the appropriate management for this group remains undetermined.

The careful selection of a relatively homogenous patient population allowed for a high degree of confidence in the interpretation of data from all of these trials. As a result, little doubt remains about the superior results of surgery over medical therapy alone in these selected patients. However, the benefits of CEA are critically dependent on the rate of perioperative complications. If the combined perioperative morbidity and mortality rate exceeds 3% in asymptomatic patients and 6% in symptomatic patients, the benefits of this procedure are quickly lost.[7] For this reason, it is critically important to ensure proper patient selection. Inclusion of patients outside of the study inclusion criteria could, theoretically, eliminate or reduce the potential benefit of treatment.

Selecting for such low-risk patients results in a considerable difference in the adverse events seen in study patients and the events seen commonly in community practice. For example, although the mortality rate in the NASCET series was 0.6%,[6] the mortality rate among Medicare beneficiaries undergoing CEA during the NASCET enrollment period was 3%.[8] In addition, the surgical results obtained by NASCET and ACAS surgeons are often not duplicated in the community. Surgical results typically are better at high-volume centers, such as study sites.[5,9] It should be noted that surgeons tend to self-report lower complication rates than independent observers, and community complication rates for CEA are often higher than the morbidity and mortality rates reported in NASCET and ACAS.[9,10] If the low complication rates in these large trials cannot be duplicated in widespread practice, the benefit of CEA may be lost. It has been estimated that for every 2% increase in the perioperative CEA complication rate, the 5-year benefit decreases by approximately 20%.[11] If the large population of patients excluded from NASCET and ACAS are unlikely to realize the benefit of CEA because of surgical morbidity, alternative therapies must be considered. These alternatives may, in fact, supplant CEA as the treatment of choice if the safety profile of these alternatives is similar to that associated with CEA.

Widespread use of CAS for the entire spectrum of carotid artery occlusive disease is neither indicated nor recommended. However, the results of early clinical series suggest that the safety of CAS is similar to that of CEA.[12-14] Because the complication rate for CAS applies to high-risk surgical candidates in most reports, certain patient subgroups considered poor candidates for CEA may benefit from CAS. Included in these subgroups are patients with one or more of the following conditions: significant coexisting medical disease, recurrent high-grade stenosis, contralateral occlusion, radiation-induced stenosis, surgically difficult-to-access high-cervical stenosis, "tandem" lesions, and intraluminal clot.

PATIENTS WITH SIGNIFICANT MEDICAL COMORBIDITIES

Every surgeon will recognize the direct relationship between clinically significant coexisting medical problems and perioperative complications associated with CEA. For years, the risk of CEA associated with medical comorbidities has been documented. This is true for nonneurologic complications, such as myocardial infarction,[15] as well as for neurologic deficits and death.[16] In an analysis of the medical complications associated with CEA, Paciaroni et al[17] found that endarterectomy was approximately 1.5 times more likely to trigger medical complications in patients with a history of myocardial infarction, angina, or hypertension. Because patients with other significant coexisting diseases were excluded from the major CEA trials, the indications for and the results of surgery in this subgroup of patients are not established. It remains important, therefore, to recognize the comorbidities that may significantly affect outcome from CEA.

Coronary artery disease is one of the most important factors when evaluating the perioperative risk of CEA.[15] The coexistence of severe carotid artery stenosis and symptomatic coronary artery disease presents the physician with a management dilemma.[17,18] The operative repair of one condition is accomplished only at substantial risk of complications from the other. In a long-term review of CEA results,[19] cardiac disease was the leading cause of death. Ironically, in an analysis of NASCET results,[20] a prior history of corrected coronary artery disease was associated with a lower CEA complication rate than was previously undiagnosed coronary artery disease. This paradox may be the result of improved cardiac and general medical care in patients undergoing treatment for coronary artery disease, many of whom may have had no regular, long-term medical care previously. Conversely, significant carotid artery disease places patients who are undergoing coronary artery bypass grafting (CABG) at increased risk for stroke, air or atheromatous embolization, or both, during cardiopulmonary bypass.[21] Faggioli et al[21] reported on a series of 539 patients undergoing CABG who underwent preoperative noninvasive evaluation (with carotid Doppler ultrasound and ocular pneumoplethysmography) for the detection of carotid artery occlusive disease. They found that a carotid artery stenosis above 75% was an independent predictor of stroke risk (odds ratio, 9.9).

In patients with significant coexistent carotid and coronary artery diseases, there is little debate that revascularization is appropriate for both conditions; however, the procedural timing introduces a clinical conundrum. Surgical options include performance of a simultaneous procedure or a staged approach in which one procedure is performed several days before the other. Published reports on combined CEA and CABG suggest that the risk of stroke or death ranges from 7.4% to 9.4%, which is roughly 1.5 to 2.0 times the risk of each operation alone.[17] Conversely, patients who undergo CEA before CABG are at highest risk for complications.[18] In this high-risk subgroup, avoiding a major operation or general anesthesia by performing angioplasty and stenting may represent a valid alternative to CEA.[22-24] Lopes et al[23] described 20 patients with unstable cardiac status who underwent CAS before CABG. One patient had a TIA, one patient developed an asymptomatic subendocardial myocardial infarction, and one patient had a groin hematoma. The mean length of stay was 14 days, and no patient had a permanent cerebrovascular event after undergoing angioplasty and stenting. This experience is in contradistinction to the results of an analysis of the English literature reported in the CEA guidelines published by the American Heart Association in which the incidence of stroke, myocardial infarction, and death is 16.44% for combined CEA and CABG; 26.15% for CEA followed by CABG; and 16.35% for CABG followed by CEA.[25] The results reported by Lopes et al[23] support the use of CAS as a valid alternative to CEA for the management of carotid artery disease in patients with coexistent symptomatic coronary artery disease that requires cardiac revascularization. In our practice, for those patients who require urgent cardiac bypass grafting, the usual poststenting antiplatelet regimen is held while the patient is receiving heparin and restarted shortly after cardiac surgery.

Other risk factors for adverse outcome in the NASCET were evaluated by Ferguson et al.[20] In their analysis of the surgical results, few clinical factors or coexisting medical conditions significantly impacted on outcome after CEA. Hemispheric rather than retinal ischemic symptoms and ipsilateral stroke on computed tomography (CT) scan imaging were associated with an increased risk of complications. Conversely, diabetes, hypertension, hyperlipidemia, age older than 65 years, symptoms within 6 months, and claudication did not effect the perioperative complication rates. The studies about medical comorbidity in carotid disease that are available to date suggest that coronary artery disease requiring CABG is the most significant medical factor affecting outcome from CEA. At our institution, CAS is recommended for patients with symptomatic coronary artery disease requiring CABG who have coexistent carotid artery stenosis measuring greater than 80% by NASCET criteria.[6]

RECURRENT CAROTID ARTERY STENOSIS

Postendarterectomy recurrent carotid artery stenosis has been increasingly recognized because long-term follow-up evaluation using noninvasive methods often is routinely performed after CEA.[26] The etiology of restenosis after successful CEA has been associated with the timing of appearance. Early recurrent stenosis, defined as restenosis occurring within 24 months after surgery, is usually caused by a myointimal fibroblastic reaction, whereas late restenosis occurs as a consequence of recurrent atherosclerotic formation.[27]

Surgical treatment of recurrent carotid artery disease poses significant challenges because dense scar tissue along the endarterectomy site renders the dissection more difficult and traumatic. In early-stage restenosis with myointimal hyperplasia, diffuse thickening of the intima and media results in fibrous hypertrophic scarring throughout the CEA site. A distinct cleavage plane between the hyperplastic lesion and the underlying media is usually impossible to identify. In late-stage recurrent atherosclerosis, the recurrent plaque is often friable and associated with intraluminal clot, which increases the risk of clot embolization during carotid artery dissection. In addition, the presence of scarring and the absence of a clear cleavage plane in the neck make exposing the carotid artery very difficult and substantially increase the risk of damage to surrounding structures. Once the carotid artery is exposed, a standard CEA is not technically feasible in many cases, and excision of the diseased segment followed by reconstruction with an interposition graft may be necessary.[26] It is not surprising, therefore, that the morbidity and mortality rates reported for surgery for carotid artery restenosis are significantly higher than those reported for primary carotid artery stenosis.[26,28]

Ideally, cases of restenosis after CEA would be treated by a procedure that does not require neck dissection or removal of the offending plaque. Angioplasty and stenting of the extracranial carotid artery is, therefore, a valid alternative to carotid artery reexploration in patients with recurrent disease. Angioplasty and stenting obviate the need for dissection, and the presence of peri-arterial scarring poses no problem because dissection is not required. By avoiding dissection through scarred tissue, cranial nerve injury, a significant problem in cases of reexploration, is eliminated.

In a report of our experience with a total of 25 endoluminal revascularization procedures performed in 21 patients with recurrent carotid artery stenosis, no major neurologic or cardiac complications occurred, and there were no deaths.[29] There was one periprocedural transient neurologic event, and one patient developed a femoral pseudoaneurysm at the access site. The mean interval from the primary CEA was 57 months (range, 8-220 months). We treated the arteries in the first seven patients in this series with angioplasty alone. However, our experience in the next 18 vessels, and the observations of others,[30-32] suggest that in this patient subgroup, the addition of stents prevents the recoil phenomenon that is observed when treating more fibrous lesions. The mean degree of stenosis, measured using the strict criteria developed by NASCET for calculation of de novo stenosis,[33] was 75% before and 9% after angioplasty with or without stenting in 24 of 25 treated vessels for which angiograms were available for review. No neurologic events occurred ipsilateral to the treated artery after a mean of 27 months in the 16 patients who underwent at least 6 months of follow-up. These early results indicate that angioplasty and stenting of carotid artery restenosis can be safely performed and that it represents a valid alternative to carotid artery reexploration procedures in this high-risk group (Fig 1).

CAROTID ARTERY STENOSIS WITH CONTRALATERAL OCCLUSION

Patients with recent symptoms referable to severe carotid artery stenosis and coexistent contralateral carotid artery occlusion face a serious prognosis. In the NASCET, the risk of ipsilateral stroke in medically treated patients with severe stenosis of the symptomatic carotid artery and occlusion of the contralateral carotid artery was 69.4% at 2 years.[34] Although CEA significantly reduced the stroke risk in this cohort of patients, the perioperative risk of stroke or death in the presence of contralateral carotid artery occlusion was 14.3%.[34] Carotid artery shunting is used in 67% to 83% of patients

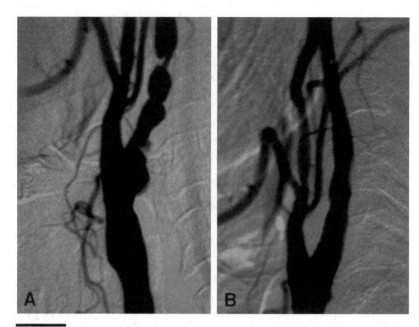

FIGURE 1.
A 68-year-old man was treated with left carotid bifurcation endarterectomy 8 years ago. Routine follow-up ultrasonography revealed progressive restenosis. Angiography before intervention **(A)** demonstrates restenosis within the region of the previous endarterectomy with significant stenosis immediately distal to the operated segment. We performed angioplasty and stenting after the administration of neuroleptanalgesia on the same day, with an excellent result **(B)**. He remains asymptomatic.

with contralateral occlusions.[34,35] However, shunt insertion may increase the risk of stroke from emboli.[36] As expected, patients with contralateral occlusions have an increased prevalence of significant risk factors, commensurate with systemic vascular disease. Combined angioplasty and stenting in this subgroup represents a valid alternative to CEA, obviating the need for temporary occlusion in the presence of reduced cerebrovascular reserve (Fig 2). In a consecutive series of 26 angioplasty and stenting procedures for carotid artery stenosis and contralateral occlusion, including 3 procedures for asymptomatic restenosis, in 23 patients at our institution during a 5-year period, no perioperative neurologic events occurred.[37] In addition, there were no strokes or cardiac events in the first month. The average ipsilateral stenosis was 78% preprocedure and 5% postprocedure. Clinical follow-up (mean, 18 months) was available for all patients but one. Nineteen patients were living

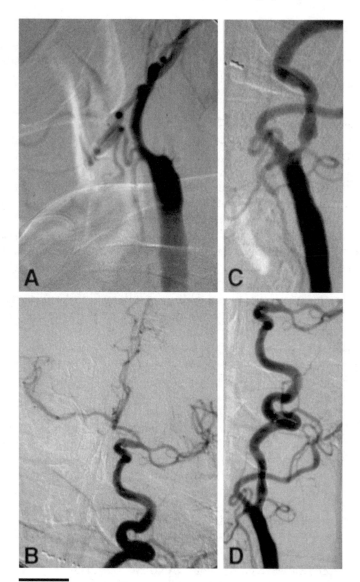

FIGURE 2.

This 67-year-old man presented with transient ischemic attacks referable to the right hemisphere. Cerebral angiography demonstrates complete occlusion of the right internal carotid artery (ICA) at its origin **(A)** with complete collateralization of flow from the left ICA **(B)**. The left cervical ICA was significantly narrowed **(C)**, and a single-photon emission computed tomographic scan confirmed hypoperfusion of the right hemisphere. Angioplasty and stenting of the left ICA improved the collateral flow and produced resolution of his symptoms **(D)**.

independently; two patients died (one of metastatic prostate carcinoma 12 months after carotid artery revascularization and the other of respiratory arrest after a prolonged hospital course and multiple complications); and one patient had a contralateral (to the treated vessel) hemispheric stroke 41 months postprocedure.

RADIATION-INDUCED CAROTID ARTERY STENOSIS

The results of human and animal studies have shown that concentrated cervical-region radiotherapy damages large arteries and leads to atherosclerosis-like occlusive disease.[38] The spectrum of the disease varies and is not dose related. As patients with head and neck malignancies survive for longer periods, radiation-induced carotid artery stenosis is sometimes observed.

Patients in whom symptomatic carotid artery occlusive disease occurs as a result of cervical radiation often require treatment because the disease progresses rapidly. Although successfully treated with direct endarterectomy or bypass of the involved arterial segments, these lesions present surgical challenges.[39] Pertinent angiographic findings include disproportionate involvement of the distal common carotid artery. Lesions are typically confined to the irradiated field and are unusually long and difficult to resect. Direct exposure of the involved carotid artery by performing standard endarterectomy is most often reported. However, most authors emphasize that a marked amount of periarterial scarring is encountered, and the planes of dissection are obscured by fibrous changes.[39] This periarterial scarring is probably related to radiation effects on the microvasculature. The wall of the artery is weakened because the vasa vasorum, which provide nutrients to the outer vessel wall, are extremely vulnerable to radiation-induced damage.[38] Infections and wound problems are increased by previous radiation treatment. Furthermore, the risk of airway obstruction can be increased in these cases.[40] The potential advantages offered by the endovascular approach for these patients are obvious.

HIGH-CERVICAL STENOSIS AND "TANDEM" LESIONS

The success of CEA is dependent on a high degree of technical perfection that may, in turn, be dependent on the ability to adequately expose the artery distal to the lesion. Accordingly, anatomic variations may increase the technical difficulty of CEA enough to negatively impact the results. A high bifurcation near the skull base, especially in a patient with a short or thick neck, or a long carotid artery stenosis that extends to the skull base can be difficult to expose surgically. Dissection of the carotid artery in these cases can be troublesome and at times extremely traumatic. These patients should be considered for stenting.

"Tandem" lesions have long been considered to be an angiographic risk factor for perioperative neurologic events.[15] The NASCET[6] excluded patients in whom intracranial lesions were more severe than surgically accessible lesions. For example, the presence of carotid siphon disease has been proposed as a contraindication to CEA because of concern of postoperative occlusion secondary to decreased flow during endarterectomy. Patients harboring such lesions may benefit from CAS because only a few seconds of occlusion time are needed to perform the procedure. If the distal stenosis is severe, angioplasty of both lesions can be performed at the same sitting. At our institution, 11 patients with tandem stenoses (two upper cervical, two petrous, six cavernous, and one supraclinoid) underwent angioplasty with and without stenting to treat carotid segment lesions.[41] The proximal lesion was considered to be the flow-limiting lesion in 10 of the 11 patients and was treated alone. In the remaining patient, both lesions were treated. No permanent neurologic events and no perioperative cardiac deficits or deaths were encountered. This experience suggests that this procedure may be a viable alternative to CEA in patients with inaccessible tandem carotid artery lesions.

CAROTID ARTERY STENOSIS WITH INTRALUMINAL CLOT

In a subgroup analysis of 53 patients enrolled in the NASCET with intraluminal clots superimposed on atherosclerotic plaque identified by angiographic procedures, the 30-day risk of stroke was 10.7% in those randomly assigned to receive medical treatment and 12% in those who underwent CEA.[42] The high morbidity rate in this subgroup is related to the presence of fresh clot and the substantial risk of emboli dislodgment during surgical dissection of the carotid artery. The use of endoluminal revascularization may be advantageous for these patients, although the safety of this approach in such cases has not been demonstrated.

Early in our experience, we used local infusion of thrombolytics before any endoluminal manipulation. In several cases, we have documented widening of the vessel lumen after local thrombolysis, which suggests clot lysis and reduction in the amount of intraluminal clot.[43] In patients who have intraluminal clot, the use of local thrombolysis before angioplasty and stenting may increase the safety of the procedure by digesting the friable portion of the thrombus, which has a higher potential for distal embolism than well-organized thrombus. More recently, we have administered antiplatelet agents to prevent thromboembolic complications, as described below. In addition to the standard preoperative use of oral antiplatelet agents, such as aspirin and ticlopidine or clopidogrel, we have used intraoperative infusion of glycoprotein IIb/IIIa inhibitors, such as abciximab (ReoPro, Centocor, Malvern, Pa) or eptifibatide (Integrilin, Cor Therapeutics, South San Francisco, Calif) to augment platelet blockade. The ability to use potent antiplatelet agents in conjunction with heparin anticoagulation during the procedure may confer an additional benefit of CAS over CEA for patients at high risk for thrombus formation. The use of distal protection devices (described in detail below) will further reduce the risk of neurologic injury from distal embolization. These devices recapitulate the process of distal occlusion and back-bleeding during CEA by permitting the surgeon to flush debris through the external carotid artery or removing it with aspiration or capture of debris.

EVALUATING AND PREPARING THE CANDIDATE FOR ANGIOPLASTY AND STENTING

Preoperative baseline neuroimaging, preferably brain magnetic resonance imaging, should be performed to document any preexisting disease and to permit comparison of preoperative and postoperative studies in the event that embolic complications are suspected. This will also rule out the presence of an intracranial process manifesting with symptoms that are indistinguishable from TIAs. Typically, noninvasive carotid duplex ultrasound studies are obtained preoperatively and postoperatively.

A complete angiographic study provides critical information regarding the presence of collateral circulation and coexistent intracranial disease that may be responsible for the clinical symptoms. In addition, intracranial views are particularly useful for baseline comparison if embolic complications happen to occur during the procedure.

Orally administered aspirin (325 mg daily) and ticlopidine (250 mg twice daily) or clopidogrel (75 mg daily) therapy are initiated 2 days before the procedure. Baseline laboratory values obtained before admission include electrolytes, serum creatinine, and blood urea nitrogen levels, and prothrombin and partial thromboplastin times. Proper informed consent is obtained. Patients are allowed to consume only clear fluids and medications starting the night before the procedure. Insulin-dependent diabetic patients receive half of their usual morning dose of insulin and are scheduled as the first case of the day. Solutions containing dextrose are used for hydration. Patients maintained on oral anticoagulation therapy discontinue its use 72 hours before the procedure and are admitted 24 hours preprocedure for heparinization. For patients with renal disease and elevated serum creatinine levels, hydration is ideally begun 24 hours before the procedure. In general, we ensure that patients are well hydrated (except those with congestive heart failure) and receive either a limited volume of contrast material or iso-osmolar contrast media.

The access site is shaved and cleansed with disinfectant solution. Distal pedal and medial tibial pulses are felt and marked for later reference, a precaution that is particularly important in elderly patients who have peripheral vascular disease. Because of the very low risk of infection after diagnostic or therapeutic endovascular procedures, prophylactic antibiotics are not routinely administered. A Foley catheter is inserted to decrease patient discomfort and restlessness as well as to allow for detailed monitoring of urinary output.

ENDOVASCULAR TECHNIQUE AND PERIOPERATIVE CARE

All patients receive a local anesthetic at the puncture site as well as intravenous hypnotic sedation and analgesic medications (ie, neuroleptanalgesia). Atropine (0.5-1.0 mg) is intravenously administered before angioplasty is performed for a stenotic lesion involving the carotid sinus (except in patients with unstable coronary disease). A premixed solution of dopamine for continuous intravenous infusion is kept immediately available in case of significant, transient hypotension. A transvenous pacemaker is immediately available should malignant bradycardia or asystole develop during balloon inflation, despite atropine administration. We do not routinely place venous sheaths before performing angioplasty. Before the introducer sheath is advanced into the common carotid artery, heparin (50 units/kg) is administered intravenously to maintain an intraoperative activated coagulation time of approximately 300 seconds throughout the procedure. In patients defined as high risk (recent symptoms or lesion length > 11.2 mm),[44] intravenous infusion of abciximab or eptifibatide is also started before crossing the lesion with the microguidewire. Infusion of the glycoprotein IIb/IIIa blocker is continued for 12 hours (abciximab) or 20 hours (eptifibatide) postoperatively.

Arterial access is usually obtained through the femoral artery. Several guidelines should be followed while gaining access to the lesion. The first is to use a guide catheter or sheath with an internal diameter sufficient to permit passage of the stent and performance of angiography with the stent in the guide catheter. This allows roadmapping and visualization of the lesion during stent or angioplasty balloon alignment. The second is to advance the guide catheter with a tapered obturator in place to reduce trauma to arterial walls. Although many devices are available, one effective procedure is to use the Cook introducer system (Bloomington, Ind) and a standard 0.035-inch hydrophilic-coated guidewire to avoid inadvertent endothelial damage during abrupt manipulation of the catheter tip. Optimum placement of the guide catheter proximal to the lesion can be arduous. This is particularly true in elderly patients in whom a tortuous, atherosclerotic aortic arch is often present. To overcome resistance to proper placement of the large guide catheter by the very tortuous origin of the great vessels from the aortic arch, navigation of the guide catheter over a very stiff wire is sometimes necessary. Catheterization of the right common carotid artery is often easier than catheterization of the left common carotid artery. Thirdly, care must be taken to avoid plaque disruption during placement of the guide catheter. We prefer to place the distal tip of a stiff guidewire into the external carotid artery to avoid additional manipulation of the internal carotid artery lesion. The introducer is removed when the guide catheter is placed in the appropriate location in the common carotid artery proximal to the lesion. Meticulous attention must be given to catheter hygiene to avoid air bubbles or thrombus formation. Heparinized saline is gently flushed through each catheter used during the procedure via a rotating hemostatic adaptor.

After guide catheter positioning, the stenosis is carefully crossed with a 0.14- to 0.18-inch microguidewire. We use a wire with a soft tip and a stiff proximal end, such as the All Star (ACS, Temecula, Calif). The wire is navigated across the lesion with the assistance of biplanar roadmap fluoroscopy. Once the wire extends through the lumen of the lesion, it is advanced past the stenosis. High-resolution biplanar digital subtraction angiography runs are performed to document stability of the lesion. Measurements of the lesion are obtained to guide further decisions regarding angioplasty balloon and stent selection. Measurements performed include lesion length as well as the diameters of the artery proximal and distal to the lesion (Fig 3).

Once satisfactory measurements have been obtained, an angioplasty balloon of appropriate size is positioned across the lesion. Balloon position is confirmed by angiography before inflation. We prefer using an oscillating balloon inflation technique in which the balloon is inflated to a pressure just below the manufacturer's

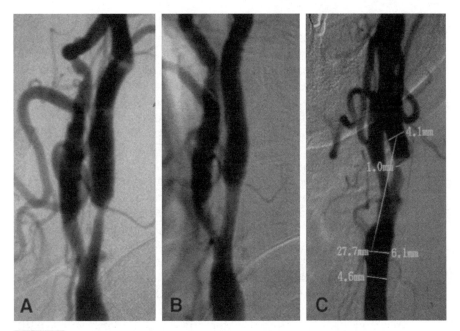

FIGURE 3.

Lateral angiography of the left common carotid artery in a symptomatic 80-year-old woman. Angiography demonstrates the significant stenosis seen in the proximal internal carotid artery before angioplasty and stenting **(A)**, and the postprocedural result **(B)**. Measurements are obtained of the normal artery proximal and distal to the lesion, lesion diameter at the point of maximal stenosis, and lesion length before crossing the lesion with a guidewire **(C)**.

recommended nominal pressure and then pressure is oscillated over 1 or 2 atmospheres for 10 to 15 seconds. We usually find that the degree of stenosis is improved after angioplasty, even when the angioplasty balloon is deliberately undersized. The most important parameters for angioplasty balloon selection are the balloon length, maximum inflation diameter, and burst pressure. In general, it is desirable to cover the entire length of the lesion with the angioplasty balloon. Placement of the balloon in arterial segments that are not diseased is avoided because this may induce intimal damage with secondary hyperplasia and arterial dissection. Ideally, the diameter of the diseased artery is reconstructed to its prediseased caliber. Overinflation of the balloon may result in intimal dissection or rupture of the balloon or artery.

Although primary stenting for carotid artery stenosis can be performed in select cases, angioplasty-assisted stenting is preferred.

The main purpose of balloon angioplasty is to facilitate stent placement. Tight stenotic lesions may be too small to primarily accept a stent. Angioplasty allows safe navigation of the relatively voluminous stent-delivery-system complex through the lesion. The angioplasty balloon is deliberately undersized to avoid overinflation and to open the artery only enough to permit passage of the stent.

Two types of stents are currently used in the carotid artery: self-expanding and balloon-expandable stents. Examples of balloon-expandable stents include the Palmaz (Johnson & Johnson Interventional Systems, Warren, NJ), which is available in several sizes that can be inflated to predetermined lengths and diameters, and the Megalink (Guidant/Advanced Cardiovascular Systems, Temecula, Calif). These stents are used infrequently because of concerns about stent collapse. The most commonly used self-expanding stent is the Wallstent (Schneider/Boston Scientific, Minneapolis, Minn). This endovascular stent has been used and approved for treatment of tracheobronchial strictures and is also available in several sizes that have a predetermined length for each diameter reached after deployment. The SMART stent (Cordis, Miami Lakes, Fla), the Acculink (Guidant), and the Memotherm (C. R. Bard, Murray Hill, NJ) use a multisegmented nickel-titanium alloy (nitinol) design that expands to a predetermined size based on its surrounding temperature at deployment. These latter stents are currently involved in Food and Drug Administration trials. Stent selection is determined by lesion length and normal arterial caliber. Stents are typically oversized by 1 to 2 mm over the arterial diameter proximal and distal to the lesion and should completely cover the lesion and a segment of normal artery proximally and distally.

Each stent has advantages and disadvantages that must be considered when choosing the most appropriate stent for each case. Balloon-expandable Palmaz stents are generally used only for short lesions because they are long and cannot be easily navigated around intravascular curves. The self-expanding Wallstent is sold premounted on its deployment device. Because of the accordion-style expansion of this stent, foreshortening occurs on deployment. As a result, distal alignment can be performed with precision before deployment, but the final position of the proximal end of the stent can be difficult to predict. Precise placement is necessary, therefore, to ensure proper coverage of the lesion. At diameters less than full expansion, a nitinol stent exerts a chronic outward force as it attempts to achieve full expansion. This may serve to maintain vessel wall apposition after deployment. Chronic outward force should be differentiated from radial force, which is the stent's ability to resist collapse after deployment and is independent of chronic outward force. After full expansion, however, this outward force is reduced to zero, and wall apposition may be lost. For this reason, nitinol stents must be slightly oversized to ensure stable placement. Frequently, there is a "waist" at the center of the stent at which the atherosclerotic lesion is generally most dense. The waist is remodeled by using postdeployment balloon angioplasty.

Serial neurologic examinations are performed after each step of the procedure involving manipulation across the stenosis to promptly recognize any changes from the patient's baseline status. After satisfactory revascularization has been achieved, final digital subtraction angiograms are obtained, including views of the ipsilateral intracranial circulation. Usually, the heparin that was administered during the procedure does not require reversal with protamine sulfate, and the femoral sheath is removed once the activated coagulation time has returned to baseline. Alternatively, in select cases including all cases maintained on abciximab or eptifibatide, we use a percutaneous closure system (Perclose, Menlo Park, Calif) that allows percutaneous suturing of the femoral arteriotomy and early mobilization of the patient. Special attention is given to the femoral artery site both before and after sheath removal to detect thrombosis or emboli in the distal leg, hematoma, or pseudoaneurysm formation.

After the procedure, patients are admitted to intensive care, and they are monitored closely for at least 18 hours. At discharge, we prescribe aspirin for patients who underwent angioplasty alone. After stenting, we prescribe ticlopidine or clopidogrel and aspirin. When ticlopidine is prescribed, a blood cell count with differential is obtained 2 weeks and 4 weeks posttreatment to detect possible ticlopidine-induced neutropenia, a potentially fatal complication.

COMPLICATION AVOIDANCE AND MANAGEMENT

Initial reports have shown the feasibility of CAS with acceptably low morbidity and mortality rates. In a review of the experience at seven centers in the United States, the results for 484 patients undergoing balloon angioplasty followed by stent deployment to treat stenosis in 543 extracranial carotid arteries were reported.[45] The stenosis was symptomatic in 56% and asymptomatic in 44%. Among the treated patients, 69% had coronary artery disease and 5.3% had contralateral carotid artery occlusion. There was a very high technical success rate (97%) and a low incidence of major strokes (3.3%).

Yadav et al[46] have detailed their results in 107 patients who underwent endoluminal revascularization procedures to treat 126 extracranial carotid arteries. In their experience, 68% of the patients had sustained a previous myocardial infarction and had undergone CABG, coronary angioplasty, or both; 77% met the NASCET exclusion criteria;[6] 9% had a contralateral carotid artery occlusion; and 11% had undergone a previous ipsilateral CEA. This series confirmed the technical feasibility of CAS and an acceptable complication rate for this procedure, considering the coexisting diseases of the treated patients. There was one case of acute stent thrombosis (0.8%). The mean stenosis was 78% ± 14% before stenting and 2% ± 5% after stenting. The minimum lumen diameter was 1.3 mm before stenting and 5.0 mm after stenting, for an acute gain of 3.7 mm. There was a single periprocedural myocardial infarction (0.9%) and a major stroke and death rate of 3%. In an update of this series,[47] the late outcome in 150 patients who underwent stenting of 180 arteries was reported: 86% of the patients had undergone either ultrasonography (24%) or follow-up angiography (62%) at 6 months. The mean stenosis was 17% ± 13%, with only 4% of the patients experiencing restenosis (defined as >50% stenosis). At follow-up, five patients required repeated angioplasty and one patient required CEA. Some degree of deformation was noted in eight stents and was considered significant only in two patients who then underwent repeated angioplasty.

These early series demonstrate that CAS can be a valid alternative to CEA in a select group of patients. However, at this time, angioplasty and stenting is neither an indicated nor a recommended treatment for patients who are good candidates for CEA because the effectiveness of the surgical procedure has already been proven. CAS is still a developing procedure that requires significant technical care and experience, similar to CEA. The safety of CAS, therefore, will be acceptable only in the most experienced hands. Unfortunately, angioplasty and stenting have been prematurely compared to CEA. As a result, a randomized trial undertaken in the United Kingdom at a single institution that compared CAS with CEA was aborted because a significant incidence of perioperative strokes was observed in the endoluminal revascularization group.[48]

When considering the effectiveness and safety of angioplasty and stenting, it is important to realize that despite the relatively low rates of mortality and major stroke, minor strokes and perioperative TIAs after endovascular treatment of carotid artery stenosis are not infrequent.[49-51] Jordan et al[50] retrospectively reviewed the complications encountered in 268 patients who underwent revascularization of 312 hemispheres, some patients having received bilateral procedures either simultaneously or at separate sessions. Minor strokes, which the authors defined as a new neurologic deficit that resolved with minimal or no deficit within 1 month of the procedure, occurred in 7.1% of patients. Perioperative TIAs occurred in 4.1%. These numbers are significant because 63% of the patients were being treated for asymptomatic carotid artery stenoses. In a preliminary report from a single center at the University of Oregon concerning 17 patients who underwent angioplasty and stenting, minor strokes (two ischemic and one hemorrhagic) occurred in 3 patients (18%).[51] All of these patients eventually recovered from their neurologic deficits. Similarly, we have identified a significant number of transient events in patients with recent symptoms and "unstable" plaques (ie, irregular lesions with or without intraluminal clot, which often produce severe stenosis causing recurrent symptoms despite antiplatelet or anticoagulant therapy). It should be emphasized that these transient events may not be detected in the absence of diligent neurologic evaluation.

The relatively high incidence of minor strokes and TIAs after CAS may be caused by microemboli. The belief that angioplasty and stent use increases the risk of thromboembolic events during the procedure is supported by research data that confirm the abundance of plaque debris liberated from the lesion during endovascular manipulation.[52,53] Théron et al[54] reported a similar embolic complication rate with patients treated with either angioplasty or direct stenting in the absence of distal protection. They concluded, therefore, that the stent provided no protection against embolization.[54] It is more likely that embolic material (plaque debris) is dislodged by stent struts moving against the vessel lumen surface. In a study in which patients undergoing CAS were compared with those undergoing CEA, the median number of cerebral emboli that were detected by transcranial Doppler study during the procedure was significantly higher in the endovascular treatment group (average, 74.0 signals).[55] The surgical group averaged 8.8 signals ($P = .0001$). Similar observations have been reported by others.[48,56-58] The endovascular maneuvers primarily associated with microemboli were those related to catheter manipulation across the plaque, prestent angioplasty, stent deployment, and postdeployment dilatation of the stent. Patients with very severe disease and a narrow lumen may be at particular risk because the balloon catheter and stent combination is invariably wider than the lumen. Most microemboli are likely lysed by endogenous fibrinolysis in the presence of adequate cerebral blood flow. A prospective study conducted in The Netherlands,[57] in which patients underwent cerebral magnetic resonance imaging before and after endoluminal revascularization, failed to demonstrate any signal intensity changes referable to emboli in 14 patients, even though two of these patients sustained perioperative neurologic events. To obviate the risk of microemboli, distal protection with a balloon system has been proposed. This approach has been pioneered by Théron et al.[59] Several manufacturers are currently working on cerebral protection by using temporary occlusion balloons or microfilters. Although balloon devices offer the ability to remove debris with an aspiration catheter, microfilters have the advantage of directly capturing debris for removal without the introduction of an additional device.

Factors associated with a higher incidence of neurologic complications include advanced age, plaque characteristics, severity of the stenosis, and the presence of tandem lesions.[60] In our experience, neurologically unstable patients, such as those with crescendo TIAs or stroke in evolution, and patients with symptomatic plaques or long lesions (>11.2 mm) are at increased risk for neurologic complications during the angioplasty and stenting procedure.[44] If an embolic complication occurs during endovascular intervention, combined superselective pharmacologic thrombolysis and mechanical thrombolysis are warranted because a spectacular result can be obtained and otherwise debilitating deficits can be reversed.[61]

RESTENOSIS AFTER ANGIOPLASTY-ASSISTED STENTING

After early experience in the coronary circulation, concerns existed regarding the long-term durability of carotid artery stents and the possible incidence of in-stent restenosis. In an early series reported by Yadav et al[46] in 81 patients, either follow-up angiograms (71 patients) or Doppler studies (10 patients) were obtained. A minor degree of myointimal hyperplasia (mean angiographic stenosis, 18% ± 12%) occurred in most patients. Hemodynamically significant restenosis (>50%) was less common, occurred in four patients (4.9%), and was not associated with clinical symptoms. Our experience supports these findings. Repeated balloon angioplasty can be performed for significant restenosis. CEA and stent removal can also be performed, although this is more technically demanding than CEA for de novo stenosis.[62]

The long-term durability of CAS is unknown. Long-term clinical follow-up is imperative. We do not perform follow-up cerebral angiography routinely in these patients because of the small but definite associated risk of complications. On the day after endoluminal revascularization, our patients undergo Doppler studies to assess baseline Doppler velocities proximal to, within, and distal to the stented segment. These studies are repeated at 3, 6, and 12 months, and yearly thereafter. Follow-up angiography is reserved for patients with increased Doppler velocities (peak systolic velocity > 200 seconds). In our experience, increased Doppler velocities do not always correlate with angiographically significant (>50%) restenosis. Differences in compliance between stented and adjacent nonstented vessel segments may produce artificially elevated Doppler velocities.

NONNEUROLOGIC COMPLICATIONS

A review of device-related technical complications is beyond the scope of this chapter but may be found in other reports that have specifically addressed this issue.[63] Nonneurologic complications include those occurring at the access site, and cardiac, renal, and hemodynamic instability.

Complications at the access site are more likely to occur in patients with peripheral vascular disease. If any resistance is encountered during advancement of the guide catheter in the femoral or iliac arteries, angiography should be performed immediately to study the anatomy.

In some cases, the coexistence of atherosclerotic disease and tortuous vessels makes navigation difficult and increases the risk of femoral artery dissections. In patients with calcified rigid vessels, compression alone is not enough to induce hemostasis at the access site after removal of the introducer sheath. Persistent hemorrhage at the access site after removal of the introducer sheath can be a harbinger of pseudoaneurysm or hematoma. Retroperitoneal hemorrhage can be fatal and is often overlooked as a cause of hemodynamic instability.[46] At our institution, the incidence of these complications has progressively decreased with experience and meticulous attention to the access site after the procedure. In addition, the availability of new percutaneous closure devices may have a significant impact on reducing these complications.

Endoluminal carotid artery revascularization is often performed in high-risk patients with significant coronary artery disease. However, the incidence of cardiac complications is relatively low because the procedure is performed after the intravenous administration of sedatives, and this avoids the need for general anesthesia. In addition, in patients with unstable angina awaiting urgent coronary revascularization, the procedure can be performed while the patient receives a continuous heparin infusion. In our recent experience, the availability of new percutaneous closure devices has eliminated the need to discontinue the heparin infusion for removal of the femoral sheath. Other authors advocate removal of the femoral sheath on the morning after the procedure to allow time for full reversal of heparin therapy.[54]

Bradycardia, hypotension, and temporary asystole related to manipulation in the region of the carotid baroceptors during angioplasty and stenting are not unusual and are clinically significant in at least 25% of patients.[50] These transient hemodynamic changes are less common when self-expanding stents are used. We recently reported an analysis of hemodynamic instability after CAS and identified factors that predict the postoperative course.[64] In a series of 51 patients treated for symptomatic (29 patients) and asymptomatic (22 patients) carotid artery stenosis, hypotension (systolic blood pressure < 90 mm Hg), hypertension (systolic blood pressure > 160 mm Hg), or bradycardia (heart rate < 60 beats/min) occurred in 22.4%, 38.8%, and 27.5% of patients, respectively. Postprocedural hypotension was predicted by intraprocedural hypotension and a history of myocardial infarction. Intraprocedural hypertension and a history of ipsilateral CEA predicted postoperative hypertension. Postprocedural bradycardia was most common after intraprocedural hypotension and bradycardia. Intensive care unit admission is mandatory after the procedure, because refractory hypotension may require treatment with continuous vasopressor infusion for titration of systolic blood pressure. Patients with critical unstable coronary artery disease are less likely to tolerate such hemodynamic changes. Whether the temporary significant hypotension observed during some of these procedures has any role in the development of postprocedural neurologic symptoms is unknown at this point.

Renal complications, although unusual, can occur in patients with renal insufficiency because of the contrast load. However, in such patients, the risk of these complications is reduced to less than the risk with open surgery and general anesthesia with proper perioperative hydration and, more recently, with the use of novel, less nephrotoxic contrast agents. Particular care must be taken to reduce the contrast load and to use diluted media for those with renal insufficiency.

SUMMARY

The relative indications for CAS versus CEA have not been determined. Whereas endarterectomy remains the gold standard for the treatment of significant carotid artery stenosis, early results suggest that angioplasty and stenting may be indicated in selected patients with risk factors for complications from endarterectomy. Despite involving vastly different mechanisms for treatment of atherosclerotic lesions, permanent neurologic morbidity and mortality rates for both techniques are similar. The transient or minor neurologic events seen more often with CAS may be amenable to prevention with distal protection techniques currently undergoing clinical testing. With careful preprocedural evaluation of medical comorbidities, appropriate treatment with antiplatelet agents, and careful evaluation of the target lesion, most potential complications of angioplasty and stenting may be avoided or at least anticipated. Further technical advancements in endovascular therapy and patient-driven preferences for less-invasive procedures are likely to expand the indications and applications of CAS.

ACKNOWLEDGMENT

We thank Paul H. Dressel for preparation of the illustrations.

REFERENCES

1. Castaneda-Zuniga WR, Formanek A, Tadavarthy M, et al: The mechanism of balloon angioplasty. *Radiology* 135:565-571, 1980.
2. Block C, Fallon JT, Elmer D: Experimental angioplasty: Lessons from the laboratory. *AJR Am J Roentgenol* 135:907-912, 1980.
3. Zollikofer CL, Salomonovitz E, Sibley R, et al: Transluminal angioplasty evaluated by electron microscopy. *Radiology* 153:372-374, 1984.
4. European Carotid Surgery Trialists' Collaborative Group: MRC European Carotid Surgery Trial: Interim results for symptomatic patients with severe (70-99%) or with mild (0-29%) carotid stenosis. *Lancet* 337:1235-1243, 1991.
5. Executive Committee for the Asymptomatic Carotid Atherosclerosis Study: Endarterectomy for asymptomatic carotid artery stenosis. *JAMA* 18:1421-1428, 1995.
6. North American Symptomatic Endarterectomy Trial Collaborators: Beneficial effect of carotid endarterectomy in symptomatic patients with high-grade stenosis. *N Engl J Med* 325:445-453, 1991.
7. Grotta J: Elective stenting of extracranial carotid arteries. *Circulation* 95:303-305, 1997.
8. Hsai DC, Krushat WM, Mmosoe LM: Epidemiology of carotid endarterectomies among Medicare beneficiaries. *J Vasc Surg* 16:201-208, 1992.
9. Faggioli GL, Curl GR, Ricotta JJ: The role of carotid screening before coronary artery bypass. *J Vasc Surg* 12:724-731, 1990.
10. Kucey DS, Bowyer B, Iron K, et al: Determinants of outcome after carotid endarterectomy. *J Vasc Surg* 28:1051-1058, 1998.
11. Hartman A, Hupp T, Koch H-C, et al: Prospective study on the complication rate of carotid surgery. *Cerebrovasc Dis* 9:152-156, 1999.

12. Chassin MR: Appropriate use of carotid endarterectomy. *N Engl J Med* 339:1468-1471, 1998.
13. Bergeron P: Carotid angioplasty and stenting: Is endovascular treatment for cerebrovascular disease justified? *J Endovasc Surg* 3:129-131, 1996.
14. Diethrich EB: Indications for carotid artery stenting: A preview of the potential derived from early clinical experience. *J Endovasc Surg* 3:132-139, 1996.
15. Joint Officers of the Congress of Neurological Surgeons and the American Association of Neurological Surgeons: Carotid angioplasty and stent: An alternative to carotid endarterectomy. *Neurosurgery* 40:344-345, 1997.
16. Sundt TM Jr, Sandok BA, Whisnant JP: Carotid endarterectomy. Complications and preoperative assessment of risk. *Mayo Clin Proc* 50:301-306, 1975.
17. Paciaroni M, Eliasziw M, Kappelle LJ, et al: Medical complications associated with carotid endarterectomy. *Stroke* 30:1759-1763, 1999.
18. Harbaugh RE, Stieg PE, Moayeri N, et al: Case problems in neurological surgery. Clinicopathological review. Carotid-coronary artery bypass graft conundrum. *Neurosurgery* 43:926-931, 1998.
19. Yashon D, Jane JA, Javid H: Long term results of carotid bifurcation endarterectomy. *Surg Gynecol Obstet* 122:517-523, 1966.
20. Ferguson GG, Eliasziw M, Barr HW, et al: The North American Symptomatic Carotid Endarterectomy Trial: Surgical results in 1415 patients. *Stroke* 30:1751-1758, 1999.
21. Faggioli GL, Curl GR, Ricotta JJ: The role of carotid screening before coronary artery bypass. *J Vasc Surg* 12:724-729, 1990.
22. Babatasi G, Massetti M, Théron J, et al: Asymptomatic carotid stenosis in patients undergoing major cardiac surgery: Can percutaneous carotid angioplasty be an alternative? *Eur J Cardiothorac Surg* 11:547-553, 1997.
23. Lopes DK, Mericle RA, Lanzino G, et al: Carotid angioplasty and stenting before coronary artery bypass grafting. *Neurosurgery* 43:686A, 1998.
24. Shawl FA: Carotid stenting in patients with symptomatic coronary artery disease: A preferred approach. *J Invas Cardiol* 10:432-442, 1998.
25. Moore WS, Barnett HJM, Beebe HG, et al: Guidelines for carotid endarterectomy: A multidisciplinary consensus statement from the ad hoc committee, American Heart Association. *Stroke* 26:188-201, 1995.
26. Meyer FB, Piepgras DG, Fode NC: Surgical treatment of recurrent carotid artery stenosis. *J Neurosurg* 80:781-787, 1994.
27. Callow AD: Recurrent stenosis after carotid endarterectomy. *Arch Surg* 117:1082-1085, 1982.
28. Hertzer NR, O'Hara PJ, Mascha EJ, et al: Early outcome assessment for 2228 consecutive carotid endarterectomy procedures: The Cleveland Clinic experience from 1989 to 1995. *J Vasc Surg* 26:1-10, 1997.
29. Lanzino G, Wakhloo AK, Fessler RD, et al: Intravascular stents for intracranial internal carotid and vertebral artery aneurysms: Preliminary clinical experience. *Neurosurg Focus* 5(4): Article 3, 1998.

30. Bergeron P, Chambran P, Benichou H, et al: Recurrent carotid disease: Will stents be an alternative to surgery? *J Endovasc Surg* 3:76-79, 1996.
31. Diethrich EB, Gordon MH, Lopez-Galarza LA, et al: Intraluminal Palmaz stent implantation for treatment of recurrent carotid artery occlusive disease: A plan for the future. *J Intervent Cardiol* 8:213-218, 1995.
32. Yadav JS, Roubin GS, King P, et al: Angioplasty and stenting for restenosis after carotid endarterectomy. Initial experience. *Stroke* 27:2075-2079, 1996.
33. North American Symptomatic Endarterectomy Trial Steering Committee: North American Symptomatic Endarterectomy Trial: Methods, patient characteristics, and progress. *Stroke* 22:711-720, 1991.
34. Gasecki AP, Eliasziw M, Ferguson GG, et al: Long-term prognosis and effect of endarterectomy in patients with symptomatic severe carotid stenosis and contralateral carotid stenosis or occlusion: Results from NASCET. *J Neurosurg* 83:778-782, 1995.
35. da Silva AF, McCollum P, Szymanska T, et al: Prospective study of carotid endarterectomy and contralateral carotid occlusion. *Br J Surg* 83:1370-1372, 1996.
36. Halsey JH Jr: Risks and benefits of shunting in carotid endarterectomy. *Stroke* 23:1583-1587, 1992.
37. Mericle RA, Kim SH, Lanzino G, et al: Carotid artery angioplasty and use of stents in high-risk patients with contralateral occlusions. *J Neurosurg* 90:1031-1036, 1999.
38. Murros KE, Toole JF: The effect of radiation on carotid arteries. A review article. *Arch Neurol* 46:449-455, 1989.
39. Loftus CM, Biller J, Hart MN, et al: Management of radiation-induced accelerated carotid atherosclerosis. *Arch Neurol* 44:711-714, 1987.
40. Francfort JW, Smullens SN, Gallagher JF, et al: Airway compromise after carotid surgery in patients with cervical irradiation. *J Cardiovasc Surg* 30:877-881, 1989.
41. Kim SH, Mericle RA, Lanzino G, et al: Carotid angioplasty and stent placement in patients with tandem stenoses. *Neurosurgery* 43:708A, 1998.
42. Villarreal J, Silva J, Eliasziw M, et al: Prognosis of patients with intraluminal thrombus in the internal carotid artery. *Stroke* 29:276A, 1997.
43. Guterman LR, Budny JL, Gibbons KJ, et al: Thrombolysis of the cervical internal carotid artery before balloon angioplasty and stent placement: Report of two cases. *Neurosurgery* 38:620-624, 1996.
44. Qureshi AI, Luft AR, Janardhan V, et al: Identification of patients at risk for periprocedural neurological deficits associated with carotid angioplasty and stenting. *Stroke* 31:376-382, 2000.
45. Iyer SS, Roubin GS, Yadav JS, et al: Angioplasty and stenting for extracranial carotid stenosis: Multicenter experience (abstract). *Circulation* 94:I-58S, 1996.
46. Yadav JS, Roubin GS, Iyer S, et al: Elective stenting of the extracranial arteries. *Circulation* 95:376-381, 1997.

47. Yadav JS, Roubin GS, Vitek J, et al: Late outcome after carotid angioplasty and stenting (abstract). *Circulation* 94:I-58S, 1996.
48. Naylor AR, Bolia A, Abbott RJ, et al: Randomized study of carotid angioplasty and stenting versus carotid endarterectomy: A stopped trial. *J Vasc Surg* 28:326-334, 1998.
49. Albuquerque FC, Teitelbaum GP, Giannotta SL: Carotid angioplasty and stenting in high-risk patients. *Neurosurgery* 43:685A, 1998.
50. Jordan WD Jr, Voellinger DC, Fisher WS, et al: A comparison of carotid angioplasty with stenting versus endarterectomy with regional anesthesia. *J Vasc Surg* 28:397-403, 1998.
51. Lutsep HL, Clark WM, Nesbit GM, et al: Angioplasty and stenting for carotid stenosis. *J Stroke Cerebrovasc Dis* 7:371A, 1998.
52. Ohki T, Marin ML, Lyon RT, et al: Ex vivo human carotid artery bifurcation stenting: Correlation of lesion characteristics with embolic potential. *J Vasc Surg* 27:463-471, 1998.
53. Théron JG, Courtheoux P, Alachkar F, et al: New triple coaxial catheter system for carotid angioplasty with cerebral protection. *AJNR Am J Neuroradiol* 11:869-877, 1990.
54. Théron JG, Buimaraens L, Coskun O, et al: Complications of carotid angioplasty and stenting. *Neurosurg Focus* 5(6):Article 4, 1998.
55. Jordan WD Jr, Voellinger DC, Doblar DD, et al: Microemboli detected by transcranial Doppler monitoring in patients during carotid angioplasty versus carotid endarterectomy. *Cardiovasc Surg* 7:33-39, 1997.
56. Ackerstaff RGA: Cerebral embolism in surgical and nonsurgical procedures of the carotid arteries. *Stroke* 29:2236A, 1998.
57. Esselink RAJ, Ernst JMPG, Overtoom TTC, et al: Neurological, transcranial Doppler and MRI monitoring in carotid stenting. *Stroke* 29:2235A, 1998.
58. Hilgertner L, Toutounchi S, Malek A, et al: Embolic signals in asymptomatic carotid primary stenosis and restenosis. *Stroke* 29:2234A, 1998.
59. Théron JG, Payelle GG, Coskun O, et al: Carotid artery stenosis: Treatment with protected balloon angioplasty and stent placement. *Radiology* 201:627-636, 1996.
60. Mathur A, Roubin GS, Iyer SS, et al: Predictors of stroke complicating carotid artery stenting. *Circulation* 97:1239-1245, 1998.
61. Hopkins LN, Lanzino G, Mericle RA, et al: Carotid intervention: A neurosurgeon's perspective. *J Invas Cardiol* 10:279-291, 1998.
62. Vale FL, Fisher WS III, Jordan WD Jr, et al: Carotid endarterectomy performed after progressive carotid stenosis following angioplasty and stent placement. Case report. *J Neurosurg* 87:940-943, 1997.
63. Holmes DR, Garratt KN, Popma J: Stent complications. *J Invas Cardiol* 10:385-395, 1998.
64. Qureshi AI, Luft AR, Sharma M, et al: Frequency and determinants of postprocedural hemodynamic instability after carotid angioplasty and stenting. *Stroke* 30:2086-2093, 1999.

CHAPTER 2

Carotid Stenting: An Interventional Vascular Surgeon's Viewpoint

Daniel G. Clair, MD
Vice Chairman, Vascular Surgery, Cleveland Clinic Foundation,
Cleveland, Ohio

As a vascular surgeon, it is difficult to heartily embrace the technology of carotid artery stent placement while knowing that the current surgical procedure to treat this problem is so successful. The extent to which carotid endarterectomy has been studied and validated in multiple trials[1-5] is unusual for a surgical procedure. Yet most practicing vascular surgeons have had patients referred for carotid artery stenting for one reason or another and have noted favorable outcomes. Even the most skeptical of surgeons would surely admit that there are certain situations in which carotid artery stenting would be preferable to standard surgical therapy because of the increased risk of endarterectomy.

It is precisely the group of high-risk surgical patients that will likely give impetus to ultimate acceptance of this technique for treating carotid artery stenosis. The high-risk surgical patients are the patients in whom initial experience with this technique has been gained by most interventionalists. And were it not for the understanding on the part of some vascular surgeons that results with certain anatomic or medical risks are not as good as those of standard risk patients, advances in the technique of carotid stenting would not have been as rapid.

Although interventionalists without any surgical expertise have performed the majority of procedures involving carotid artery stent placement, it is only the interventional surgeon that can render an unbiased recommendation for the best therapy for the patient. When the physician caring for the patient performs all the available therapies and understands the risks and benefits associated with them, he can, without bias, make a recommendation to the patient. The interventional surgeon as well can offer combinations of therapy, which might otherwise be unavailable. Clearly, vascular surgeons need to be involved in performing carotid stent procedures and in ensuring that trials designed to evaluate the safety and efficacy of this therapeutic modality are rigorous, safe, and generate reliable data that will help us to treat our patients better. With the current technique of carotid endarterectomy, risks are very low, and it is clear that carotid stenting will have a difficult time matching the outcomes of the best surgeons performing a procedure perfected over the last several decades. Yet it is not truly the interventionalist's experience alone that will ultimately advance the technique of carotid stenting. As the technology for performing this procedure improves based on recommendations of experienced technicians, it is likely that the technique will match or potentially even surpass the results achieved with carotid endarterectomy.

Vascular surgeons should remain skeptical of single-institution reports on outcomes of carotid stenting, but we should also recognize the importance of the technological advances that are being made in devices used for carotid artery stenting.

This chapter presents the approach to the patient with carotid stenosis, with special emphasis on assessing patients for appropriateness for recommending carotid artery stenting; selecting patients for carotid stenting; assessing patient risk for interventional therapy for carotid stenosis; reviewing techniques for carotid stenting; and assessing carotid artery stent outcomes from a surgeon's perspective.

APPROACH TO THE PATIENT WITH CAROTID STENOSIS

The majority of vascular surgeons evaluating patients for carotid surgery make use of noninvasive testing to assess the extent of disease in the cervical carotid artery. Although duplex evaluation of the carotid artery is important in assessing whether a patient has significant carotid occlusive disease, it is not the only basis on which decisions for carotid surgery are made. Depending on the presence or absence of symptoms, the severity of the stenosis, the age, and comorbid risks factors, a decision is made to recommend either continued observation or carotid revascularization. For the time being, most patients will continue to be recommended for surgical therapy for this problem. But surgical therapy is not the only method of revascularizing the carotid artery, and there are clearly subgroups of patients for whom surgical therapy has higher risk. Those patients at higher risk ought to have a frank discussion with their physician about what all the alternatives for therapy are, including medical therapy. This discussion should also include a discussion regarding carotid stenting.

In a recent review of prospectively collected registry data, more than 3000 patients undergoing carotid endarterectomy at the Cleveland Clinic[6] were evaluated and stratified into either high-risk or low-risk categories based on the presence or absence of one or more of the following: coronary artery disease requiring angioplasty or bypass within the last 6 months, history of congestive heart failure, severe chronic obstructive pulmonary disease, or renal insufficiency with a serum creatinine level greater than 3.0 mg/dL. In the 594 patients meeting the criteria to be classified as high risk, the composite end point of stroke/myocardial infarction or death occurred in 7.4% during the index hospitalization. This was significantly higher than the rate of 2.9% in the low-risk group ($P < .0005$). Single-event evaluation of stroke (3.5% vs 1.7%) and death (4.4% vs 0.3%) were statistically elevated as well in the high-risk group. Even excluding the patients undergoing combined carotid and coronary procedures, the composite end point evaluation revealed less favorable outcomes in the high-risk group.

A number of factors have traditionally been associated with higher risk for patients undergoing carotid endarterectomy. These high-risk markers include symptomatic lesions, advanced age, severe cardiac or pulmonary disease, renal insufficiency, diabetes, prior carotid endarterectomy, prior neck irradiation, prior radical neck dissection, contralateral carotid occlusion, and fluctuating findings on neurologic examination. Although many institutional series have looked at these issues separately and documented excellent results,[7-16] these subgroups have been recognized as having less satisfactory results when evaluated in multi-institutional trials.[17-19] Because of concerns regarding outcomes in these patients, a large number of these patient characteristics were exclusion criteria for large randomized trials.[1,3,5]

By using currently available predictors of higher risk patients and by correlating these characteristics with personal or group outcome data, nearly all surgeons should be able to isolate patients in their practices in whom the risk for surgery is increased. It is in this high-risk group of patients that initial evaluation of carotid stenting seems warranted. At the very least, these patients can and should be safely enrolled in randomized trials comparing carotid stenting with surgery, or enrolled in high-risk carotid stenting registries if the patients are deemed too high risk for surgery. Currently, stenting is offered to patients with severe cardiopulmonary disease, contralateral carotid occlusion, age greater than 80 years, contralateral recurrent nerve injury, prior radiation therapy, prior carotid endarterectomy, and severe tandem carotid lesions. Ongoing high-risk trials include the SAPPHIRE trial subsidized by Cordis (Johnson & Johnson, Warren, NJ) and the ARCHER trial subsidized by Guidant (Guidant, Menlo Park, Calif). Each of these randomized high-risk trials also includes a high-risk registry for patients not felt to be surgical candidates and includes the use of a protection device. With the initiation of the CREST trial, we will hopefully also soon begin randomization for the group of patients with symptomatic high-grade carotid stenosis, another high-risk group. Although the trial currently does not include the use of a cerebral protection device, it is hoped that with proven safety and efficacy of a device, its use can be included in the trial.

Choosing patients to offer carotid stenting also requires a clear understanding of the clinical characteristics that make a patient at high risk. These risk factors include advanced age, large clinical stroke, changing findings on neurologic examination, or absent femoral pulses. These risk factors should be evaluated in conjunction with the patient's surgical risk for endarterectomy and the experience of the interventionalist.

Once a patient is to undergo carotid stenting, antiplatelet therapy is initiated with both aspirin, 325 mg once daily, and clopidogrel (Plavix, Sanofi Winthrop, New York, NY), 300 mg loading dose and 75 mg once daily. These medications are continued through the time of the procedure. In addition, arch and carotid arteriography is necessary before proceeding with carotid stenting. This evaluation will help to assess the anatomic risk factors the patient possesses. Anatomical criteria that add potential risk to this procedure include a severely calcified, atherosclerotic arch, severely tortuous arch vessels, a markedly rotated arch with vessel origins markedly below the peak of the aortic arch, proximally located common carotid stenoses, heavily calcified circumferential lesions, and a thrombus located in the carotid lesion. If the patient understands that high-risk anatomy may preclude continuing with stenting, diagnostic studies and therapeutic intervention can be performed at the same time. A thorough preoperative neurologic assessment is helpful to ensure that the interventionalist is familiar with the patient's preexisting limitations. A preprocedural computed tomography scan of the head as well will allow the identification of preexisting anatomical abnormalities. Patients are informed beforehand that they will not receive sedation during the procedure so that neurologic status can be assessed. Antiplatelet therapy as described above is confirmed. The patient will need large-bore intravenous access should volume resuscitation be needed. Headstraps for positioning can induce anxiety. The use of a head cradle cushion is favored for head positioning. Continuous electrocardiographic and oxymetric monitoring is performed routinely. All patients have continuous intra-arterial pressure monitoring via the access sheath. Noninvasive blood pressure monitoring is also carried out for times during which the pressure cannot be measured through the sheath.

TECHNIQUE OF CAROTID STENTING

Many of the risks associated with intra-arterial procedures are related to the access. Care at each point at which problems occur can alleviate later difficulties. Avoidance of arterial access above the inguinal ligament or below the common femoral bifurcation will limit the potential for later problems. Routine access with a 5-French sheath is obtained, and if selective views of the arch anatomy and carotid arteries have not been obtained, a pigtail flush catheter is passed into the ascending aorta where a 30° left anterior oblique view is obtained. In situations where the arch is more rotated, the obliquity of this view can be increased. The arch view is used as a map to assist with obtaining access to the origins of the carotid arteries.

Gaining access to the carotid arteries is dependent on using the correct catheter for the anatomy. Using a less angled catheter allows easier tracking along the wire into the common carotid artery. If possible, an angled Glide Catheter (Boston Scientific Corp, Watertown, Mass) is used to access the origins of the innominate and left common carotid arteries. Where increased angulation at the origins of these vessels is noted, the choice of catheter might include the H1H (Angiodynamics, Queensbury, NY), Judkins right 4, or internal mammary catheter. With further angulation at the origin seen usually where the vessels arise closer to the ascending aorta, a reverse curved catheter may be necessary. The VTK catheter (Cook Inc, Bloomington, Ind) possesses an angle that makes it well suited to gain access to the arch vasculature. In addition, one may use the Sos catheter (Angiodynamics, Queensbury, NY) or Simmons 1, 2, or 3 catheters (Merit Medical, Angleton, Tex). The larger Simmon's catheters have the potential for increasing embolization because the catheters require reforming in the arterial system, sometimes even at the aortic valve. Access with the less curved catheters is best obtained by initially advancing the catheter beyond the vessel in question. The catheter can then be rotated in a clockwise direction to allow the tip to lay flat across the top of the aortic arch. While the catheter is slowly being retracted, slow counterclockwise rotation should be performed to allow the catheter tip to engage the vessel orifice. This technique tends to work very well with the nonreversed curve catheters. Care needs to be taken with the catheters with a slightly larger angle, such as the JR4 (Cordis Corp, Miami, Fla) and the IMA (Merit Medical). The reversed curve catheters are best formed distal to the arch vessels if possible. The catheter is then advanced across the arch to engage the orifice of the desired vessel. Should the catheter progress beyond the desired orifice, clockwise rotation to "flatten" the catheter out in the arch or even further to allow the tip of the catheter to aim toward the base of the arch allows retraction without the tip of the catheter dragging across vessel wall.

Once the orifice of the vessel has been engaged, the vessel is cannulated with the use of the 0.035-in stiff, angled Glide Wire (Boston Scientific). Care is taken to ensure the wire stays below the lesion in question. With the wire stabilized, the catheter is advanced into the common carotid artery. Although the less curved catheters often follow the wire without much difficulty, the reversed curved catheters require more patience to advance. In some instances, the catheter needs to be exchanged over the wire to allow a less angled catheter to be advanced. Care should be taken to keep the wire monitored during catheter exchanges because the wire can easily be dislodged during this maneuver. In some instances, the wire may need to be advanced into the right subclavian artery to allow catheter exchange without losing wire access. In difficult situations, one might need to advance the wire into the external carotid artery to advance the catheter.

Once the catheter is positioned within the carotid artery, its position ought to be confirmed with contrast injection under fluoroscopy. This will ensure that there is no dissection and that the catheter is in the appropriate vessel. Care should be taken when removing a wire from a catheter in the carotid circulation because rapid removal of the wire can lead to the intrainment of air and air embolization. The wire should be removed slowly or with a flush of saline over the hub of the catheter to prevent this occurrence. When the position of the catheter is confirmed, the patient is systemically heparinized with a target activated clotting time (ACT) of 220 to 250 seconds. The angled Glidewire is then advanced into the external carotid artery. This maneuver is performed under road mapping guidance, and the catheter is advanced into the external carotid artery over the wire. The Glidewire is then exchanged for an exchange length 0.035-in Amplatz super stiff wire (Cook) with a 1-cm flexible tip. This wire will allow the sheath to access the common carotid artery.

A 7-French, 90-cm Shuttle (Cook) sheath is then advanced into the common carotid artery over the Amplatz wire. The side arm of the sheath can be connected to a manifold, which should allow continuous intra-arterial pressure monitoring. Adequate access to the common carotid artery is necessary because premature withdrawal of the sheath can have catastrophic consequences. The extra time taken to ensure the sheath is well positioned in the common carotid artery is well worth it.

When the carotid lesion precludes access to the external carotid artery with the stiff wire, one may need to attempt access with the rigid wire within the common carotid artery below the lesion. With very tortuous anatomy and inaccessibility of the external carotid artery for the rigid wire, careful consideration should be given to changing the plan for the patient to surgery. For the interventional surgeon, this change of plans should not induce any sense of anxiety because the goal is for the safest procedure for the patient.

The imaging equipment is then positioned in the most favorable position to allow visualization of the stenosis at maximum. It is also helpful to avoid any overlying external branches, which may obscure the view of the lesion. Foreign objects interfering with the image, as well, should be removed. This should include removal of hearing aids, jewelry, and dental prostheses if they have not already been removed. A steerable 0.014 or 0.018-in wire is then shaped appropriately and advanced in an atraumatic fashion across the lesion. The wire is positioned distally at the skull base. The wire choice depends on available equipment and the anatomy both proximal and distal to the lesion, as well as the nature of the lesion itself. Frequently, the predilation balloon is already loaded on the wire to save time. The inner lumen of the balloon is matched to the wire used to limit any ledge as the balloon crosses the lesion. A 4.0-mm balloon diameter is appropriate for most lesions. For extremely tight lesions, a preliminary dilatation with a 2.0-mm, low-profile coronary balloon is helpful. Inflation and deflation of the balloon should be performed cautiously. Slow deflation of this balloon may decrease the rate and number of microemboli.

Imaging of the lesion after predilatation will give the operator an assessment of whether the lumen is large enough to allow passage of the stent delivery system. Occasionally, in heavily calcified lesions, additional dilation will need to be done with a 5-mm balloon.

For most lesions, a self-expanding stent appropriately sized to the artery should be chosen. Options currently available to interventionalist performing this procedure with commercially available products include the Wallstent (Boston Scientific), the SMART stent (Cordis), the Memotherm Flex stent (Angiomed Bard Inc, Kartsruh, Germany), and the Dynalink stent (Guidant). Balloon-expandable stents can be useful in extremely high lesions because self-expanding delivery systems placed distally in the internal carotid artery can cause significant damage. Stent length should be chosen such that there will be adequate length of the stent above and below the lesion to stabilize the stent. One should not attempt to size the length of the stent to exactly cover the lesion. The orifice of the external carotid artery can be crossed with the stent, and commonly, as most surgeons know, the lesion extends to the origin of the internal carotid artery even though this may not be evident from the angiographic image. The stent is advanced across the lesion and then retracted into appropriate position.

The distal first several millimeters of the stent should be deployed slowly initially and allowed to expand fully and stabilize against the arterial wall beyond the lesion. After this initial placement, the stent is fully deployed slowly through the lesion. Especially with the nitinol stents, time should be allowed before withdrawing the delivery system because the stent will expand after initial deployment. This additional time can avoid potential catching of the delivery system on the stent. This withdrawal should always be performed under fluoroscopic guidance to ensure the devices are moving freely. Despite the appearance of adequate expansion of the stent, all stents should be postdilated with either a 5- or 6-mm-diameter balloon whose length is no longer than the stent deployed. No attempt should be made to dilate the artery to its full diameter. Aggressive dilation can lead to increased embolic events.

Frequently, the balloon chosen will be of a shorter length than the stent to allow for inflation within the stent to prevent potential dissection, which can complicate balloon inflation outside the stent. If for some reason the balloon must extend beyond the limits of the stent, additional balloon length should extend proximally. Distal dissections in the internal carotid can be very troublesome and difficult to correct. Balloon inflation and especially deflation if possible should be done slowly to attempt to limit embolization potential. The patient should be carefully observed during all inflations to assess neurologic status and to ensure that the typical bradycardic response to carotid dilatation can be recognized and treated early. Patients with contralateral occlusion can be observed for loss of consciousness or seizure activity. Atropine, dopamine, and pressure infusion devices are mandatory components of the interventional room inventory. Early dosing with 0.5 mg of atropine can limit the bradycardia some patients experience. Removal of the balloon should be performed carefully because the balloon can tend to catch on the stent interstices. Should this occur, full deflation should be confirmed. The balloon may need to be advanced gently to free it. Normally with patience and attention to detail, the balloon is removed with no impingement.

Completion arteriography of the target lesion and intracranial circulation should be performed to assess the early postintervention status of these vessels. On completion of stenting, attention should be turned to sealing the access site. Any of the available closure devices can be used for this purpose, or the ACT can be allowed to return to near normal and the sheath removed using direct pressure. Patients should remain in a closely monitored setting for at least the next 4 to 8 hours. Frequent neurologic monitoring and careful attention to the blood pressure is mandatory. Currently, patients remain in a telemetry setting for the night after the procedure.

Mention should be made of technique modifications that can be made with smaller devices that are currently under investigation. These devices, Precise stent (Cordis) and Acculink stent (Guidant), have reduced the size of sheath necessary for delivery to 6 French. These stents can also be delivered with the use of formed guides. The use of guide catheters for delivery of devices is much more familiar to cardiologists because this technique is what is used mostly for coronary interventions. The guide catheter can be passed into the common carotid artery over the diagnostic catheter, and often this can be done without wire access to the external carotid artery. Although this technique is at times helpful, the guides can be stiffer than currently available flexible sheaths and difficult to advance into the common carotid artery in an atraumatic fashion. It is helpful to be familiar with both techniques so that the most advantageous technique can be used in the appropriate situation.

Protection devices further alter the basic technique, but their use will not be covered in this chapter, since clear proof of efficacy and safety await continued trials.

OUTCOME OF CAROTID STENTING

It is impossible to know at this point what the precise outcome of carotid stenting should be; however, a review of currently available data can provide significant information regarding outcomes.

Although most surgeons remain somewhat skeptical, the technique continues to evolve, and outcomes will continue to improve. Surgical and medical community skepticism is aggravated by personal communications from interventionalists claiming a complete lack of adverse neurologic events. And although the difference between major and minor strokes are significant, surgical therapy has been judged by the standard of any stroke. Despite the roadblocks to acceptance of this technique, increasing numbers of these procedures are being performed, with at least one center in this country claiming to have performed well over 1000 carotid stent procedures. Lower profile stent delivery systems, cerebral protection devices, and increasing operator experience will make results in the near future better than what we have available currently. Results of the trials currently underway are eagerly awaited. Data available reveal that although the technique has limitations, the results are clearly better than the initial published data.

Recent published series are presented in Table 1. These results are reported based on data from the most experienced centers in the world. Wholey et al[21] reviewed the data from a registry incorporating data from Europe, North and South America, and Asia. The results of this registry are impressive, and the number of cases shows the rate at which this procedure is beginning to be performed. Most of these cases have been performed without protection devices or the miniaturized technology that could even further improve the outcomes of this procedure.

The only available study comparing stenting with surgery is the CAVATAS study. Although the final published trial data are awaited, we do know preliminarily that the two procedures were similar in outcomes; however, the combined stroke/mortality rate was excessively high (10.3%) in the surgery group. Arguably, the same could be said of interventional results, with a combined stroke/mortality rate of 10.4%. Many of the interventional patients were treated with angioplasty alone with stenting reserved. Experience has shown that this form of therapy will increase the stroke risk.

Although the final outcome of trials will determine how patients will be treated in the future, it is clear that the patients are ultimately the beneficiaries. There are certainly patients for whom the morbidity of carotid endarterectomy is high. The best example of these patients are those who have had radical neck surgery and prior radiation therapy. Those who have operated on these patients know that there will likely be at least a group of patients for whom this procedure is a significant advance. In addition, the technological development of low-profile stents will be of benefit

TABLE 1.
Results of Carotid Stenting

Author	Year	No. of Patients	No. of Lesions	Technical Success	Major Stroke	Minor Stroke	Death	30-Day Combined Stroke Mortality
Mathias[20]	1999	633	799	99%	1.1%	1.6%	0.3%	3%
Wholey[21]	2000	4757	5210	98.4%	1.49%	2.72%	0.86%	5.07%
Dangas[22]	2000	133	140	99.3%	0.9%	5.3%	0.7%	6.9%
Roubin[23]	2001	528	604	98%	1%	4.8%	1.6%	7.4%
Bergeron[24]	1999	99	99	97%	0	1%	0	1%

in the periphery and will allow even less morbid interventions elsewhere in the arterial system for occlusive disease.

Surgeons have been instrumental in advancing less invasive methods of treating other types of traditionally surgical problems. Carotid stenting is no exception. With appropriate caution, the majority of surgeons strive to provide for their patients the least morbid therapy for their disease. With surgeons as interventionalists and heavily invested in the performance of this procedure and trials evaluating it, we can be assured that the results of these trials will be ones that we can point to for our patients to help them make decisions regarding care.

REFERENCES

1. North American Symptomatic Carotid Endarterectomy Trial Collaborators: Beneficial effect of carotid endarterectomy in symptomatic patients with high-grade carotid stenosis. *N Engl J Med* 325:445-453, 1991.
2. Barnett HJM, Taylor DW, Eliasziw M, et al: Benefit of carotid endarterectomy in patients with symptomatic moderate or severe stenosis. *N Engl J Med* 339:1415-1425, 1998.
3. European Carotid Surgery Trialists' Collaborative Group: MRC European Carotid Surgery Trial: Interim results for symptomatic patients with severe (70-99%) or with mild (0-29%) carotid stenosis. *Lancet* 337:1235-1243, 1991.
4. European Carotid Surgery Trialists' Collaborative Group: Endarterectomy for moderate symptomatic carotid stenosis: Interim results from the MRC European Carotid Surgery Trial. *Lancet* 347:1591-1593, 1996.
5. Executive Committee for the Asymptomatic Carotid Atherosclerosis Study: Endarterectomy for asymptomatic carotid artery stenosis. *JAMA* 273:1421-1428, 1995.
6. Ouriel K, Hertzer NR, Beven EG, et al: Pre-procedural risk stratification: Identifying an appropriate group in whom to study the role of carotid stenting. *Circulation* 100:I-67, 1999.
7. Hill BB, Olcott C IV, Dalman RL, et al: Reoperation for carotid stenosis is as safe as primary carotid endarterectomy. *J Vasc Surg* 30:26-35, 1999.
8. O'Hara PJ, Hertzer NR, Mascha EJ, et al: Carotid endarterectomy in octogenarians: Early results and late outcome. *J Vasc Surg* 27:860-871, 1998.
9. Hoballah JJ, Nazzal MM, Jacobonicz C, et al: Entering the ninth decade is not a contraindication for carotid endarterectomy. *Angiology* 49:275-278, 1998.
10. Hamdan AD, Pomposelli FB Jr, Givvons GW, et al: Renal insufficiency and altered postoperative risk in carotid endarterectomy. *J Vasc Surg* 29:1006-1011, 1999.

11. Sternbergh WC III, Garrard CL, Gonze MD, et al: Carotid endarterectomy in patients with significant renal dysfunction. *J Vasc Surg* 29:1006-1011, 1999.

12. Akbari CM, Pomposelli FB Jr, Gibbons GW, et al: Diabetes mellitus: A risk factor for carotid endarterectomy? *J Vasc Surg* 25:672-677, 1997.

13. Ballotta E, Da Giau G, Guerra M: Carotid endarterectomy and contralateral internal carotid artery occlusion: Perioperative risks and long-term stroke and survival rates. *Surgery* 123:234-240, 1998.

14. Coyle KA, Smith RB III, Salam AA, et al: Carotid endarterectomy in patients with contralateral carotid occlusion: Review of a 10-year experience. *Cardiovasc Surg* 4:7175, 1996.

15. Adelman MA, Jacobowitz GR, Riles TS, et al: Carotid endarterectomy in the presence of a contralateral occlusion: A review of 315 cases over a 27-year experiences. *Cardiovasc Surg* 3:307-312, 1995.

16. Tretter MJ Jr, Hertzer NR, Mascha EJ, et al: Perioperative risk and late outcome of nonelective carotid endarterectomy. *J Vasc Surg* 30:618-631, 1999.

17. Rothwell PM, Slattery J, Warlow CP: Clinical and angiographic predictors of stroke and death from carotid endarterectomy: Systematic review. *BMJ* 315:1571-1577, 1997.

18. Sundt TM Jr, Houser OW, Sharbrough FW, et al: Carotid endarterectomy: Results, complications and monitoring techniques. *Adv Neurol* 16:97-119, 1977.

19. Hsia DC, Krushat WM, Moscoe LM: Epidemiology of carotid endarterectomies among Medicare beneficiaries. *J Vasc Surg* 16:201-208, 1992.

20. Mathias K, Jager H, Sahl H, et al: Interventional treatment of arteriosclerotic carotid stenosis. *Radiology* 39:125-134, 1999.

21. Wholey MH, Wholey M, Mathias K, et al: Global experience in cervical carotid artery stent placement. *Cathet Cardiovasc Interv* 50:160-167, 2000.

22. Dangas G, Laird JR Jr, Satler LF, et al: Postprocedural hypotension after carotid artery stent placement: Predictors and short- and long-term clinical outcomes. *Radiology* 215:677-683, 2000.

23. Roubin GS, New G, Iyer S, et al: Immediate and late clinical outcomes of carotid artery stenting in patients with symptomatic and asymptomatic carotid artery stenosis: A 5-year prospective analysis. *Circulation* 103:532-537, 2001.

24. Bergeron P, Becquemin JP, Jausseran JM, et al: Percutaneous stenting of the internal carotid artery: The European CAST I Study. Carotid Artery Stent Trial. *J Endovasc Surg* 6:155-159, 1999.

PART II

Aortic Disease

CHAPTER 3

Current Situation on Stenting for Aortic Aneurysms: The European Experience

P. R. F. Bell, MB, ChB, MD, FRCS
Professor of Surgery, University of Leicester, Leicester Royal Infirmary, Leicester, England

Abdominal aortic aneurysms are a significant cause of mortality in the Western world and are present in about 5% of men older than 65 years.[1] They are frequently asymptomatic and are thought to be responsible for many thousands of deaths each year when they rupture. Historically, these lesions have been discovered incidentally either by X ray or by clinical examination when they become tender. More recently, with the increasing use of ultrasound as a nonspecific abdominal investigation for pain, many more are being diagnosed before they rupture. In addition, clinical trials now under way will provide evidence on the importance of screening, which is likely to become routine in the future.

Abdominal aortic aneurysms have historically been treated by open surgery. Since the 1950s, results have been excellent in general, with mortality rates of approximately 6% in multicenter studies[2] and rates as low as 2% in specialized centers,[3] particularly if risk factors are taken into consideration. Open surgery is therefore a safe and durable operation that is suitable for most patients who have no morbidity (American Society of Anaesthetists [ASA] Score 1, 2, or 3). In 1988, Volodos et al[4] used endovascular techniques (EVAR) to insert the first stent-supported graft into a saccular thoracic aneurysm with success, and in 1991, Parodi et al[5] popularized this technique in patients with aortic aneurysms. Since then, many thousands of these grafts have been inserted, and there are now a number of different devices that can be used to treat patients with an aortic aneurysm. With the availability of a good open technique, one has to ask why it is necessary to try and improve matters. The general trend towards minimally invasive surgery has resulted in its becoming a necessity, as more and more patients demand this type of treatment. Of course, if this procedure causes less morbidity and mortality than an open operation, then clearly a smaller incision with a shorter hospital stay and recovery period will be beneficial to all concerned.

Opinions will vary widely about which aneurysms to treat. Some surgeons would advocate that aneurysms as small as 4 cm need treatment, whereas others would say that they should not be dealt with until they reach 6 cm or more. In this context, the small aneurysm–randomized study carried out in the United Kingdom was an important indicator of which lesions should be treated.[6] This study showed that if the aneurysm is less than 5.5 cm in diameter, the risk of rupture and death is no more than if surgery is undertaken, with being approximately 1% per year. One concern of the trial was that patients were operated on when the aneurysm reached 5.5 cm in diameter. It may be that they could have been left for longer before surgery was undertaken. Clearly, the results of endovascular treatment will depend on the fitness of the patient for surgery and on the size of the lesion being treated. Small aneurysms are very easy to treat by endovascular methods, the risks are small, and any results that are produced in the absence of a randomized trial have to be assessed in the light of that knowledge. Many large series contain lesions of this type. It is likely that patients who have small aneurysms will have fewer complications and recover more quickly after endovascular repair at least in the short term, than will those with large aneurysms with wide necks.

Before this treatment is used more widely, however, a number of issues have to be resolved. The first and most obvious one is that endovascular repair has not been compared with standard treatment, which must remain the gold standard and is known to work well even though it has perhaps not been exposed to as rigorous a follow-up as it might have been. We need to know the answer to many questions before a feasibility study slips into routine clinical practice so common in surgery. In this context, we need to know which aneurysms to treat, about relative mortality, the complications, durability of the graft, the costs involved, and the effect on the quality of life in terms of follow-up and other additional treatments that might become necessary.

MORTALITY

The mortality rate after endovascular procedures should in theory be less than that for open surgery, because the main cause of mortality is aortic clamping. Even in the hands of technically adept surgeons, the aorta will be clamped for approximately 30 minutes. By comparison, the insertion of a stent takes only a few minutes at most, and the relative strain on the heart must be much less. In spite of this, the mortality rates of the two procedures are similar. In a recent publication from the RETA (Registry for Endovascular Treatment of Aneurysms in the United Kingdom), the overall mortality rate for patients undergoing endovascular repair was 7%.[7] This rate is similar to those found in the majority of multicenter trials on open repair. The Eurostar Registry, which contains more patients, has reported an overall perioperative death rate of 3.2%.[8] The difference in these two registries is that patients with more comorbidities (ASA Score 4 or 5) were treated in the RETA group, in which uni-iliac grafts tended to be used to treat unfit patients (Fig 1). The message from these two publications is that the mortality rate for endovascular repair compared with that for open repair in fit patients is not very different.

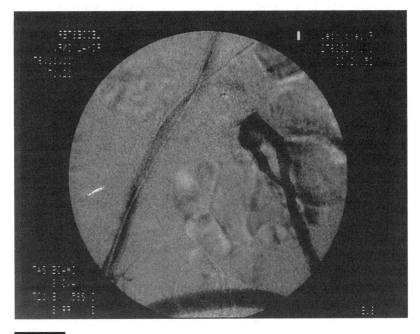

FIGURE 1.
An aorto-uni-iliac graft, useful in ruptures and difficult cases.

In unfit patients in whom surgery is usually not undertaken, the mortality rate is relatively high for endovascular repair (approximately 18%), but patients who have open surgery do have a higher mortality rate than this.

Many centers report very low overall mortality rates, but it is difficult to know what this means because many patients with small aneurysms may have been treated. Until we can compare the same kind of patients in each treatment group, we will not be in a position to say what the comparative mortality rates are. However, the mortality rates would have to be very low indeed to improve on those seen with open operations when fit patients are dealt with. It would seem that the mortality rates are comparatively best for those patients who are unfit for open repair or in whom a mortality rate of 20% to 30% might be expected. These patients include those who are unfit because of cardiac disease or who may have severe respiratory disease. One intriguing question is whether the other problems affecting these patients will lead to their death long before the aneurysms rupture, making repair unnecessary. At the moment, large numbers of such patients are being dealt with in Europe. Therefore, it currently can be concluded that the mortality rates for open repair versus endovascular treatment may not be very different, and for unfit patients they may be quite high.

IMMEDIATE SURGICAL INSULT

There is little doubt that the use of an endovascular device imposes much less insult to the patient. Such patients are usually able to go home in 2 or 3 days and do not necessarily need intensive therapy unit care. They have less wound pain and fewer respiratory complications,[9] and can usually resume their normal activities much more quickly. There is a good deal of biochemical evidence that the trauma caused by EVAR is significantly less than that imposed by open repair. For example, the blood levels of cytokines such as interleukin (IL)–6 and IL–8 are lower with endovascular repair, and the markers of potential renal damage and white blood cell activation are also reduced.[10,11] In addition, such patients do not have other potentially serious problems associated with open repair such as gastrointestinal upset, wound infections, herniation, adhesions, and wound pain. Patients who have had open repair often require 3 months to return to their level of preoperative activity. The short-term comparison therefore is not in question, and there is no doubt that an endovascular procedure has a much shorter recovery period. However, this has to be weighed against the long-term outlook. In conclusion, endovascular repair is less traumatic in the immediate postoperative phase, but this is not projected into a lower morbidity.

DURABILITY

One of the main problems related to endografting is whether or not the graft, held in place as it is by a metal stent, will stay there. We now know that incorporation of the graft into the aortic wall does not occur.[12] However, if bare metal stents are placed above the graft, these do get covered by endothelium and become rigidly adherent to the aortic wall. This occurrence has implications for stent design in the future. We also know that the neck of the aorta above the aneurysm dilates by 1 to 2 mm a year (Fig 2).[13] With time, this dilatation may eventually lead to the stent graft falling out of the neck unless it is incorporated, which at present does not appear to significantly occur. A recent, as yet unpublished study, suggests that when balloon-expanded stents are used (the Palmaz stent) after initial neck enlargement from oversizing, the neck stops expanding. If, however, a self-expanding stent is used, perhaps by exerting continuing force on the vessel wall, the neck of the aneurysm continues to expand. This again has implications for stent-graft design. It may be that some form of fixation with hooks

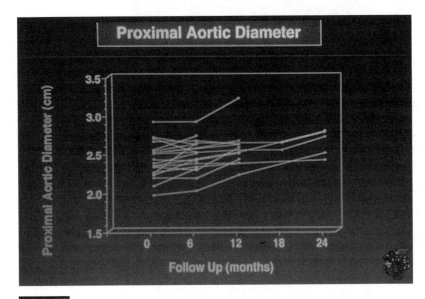

FIGURE 2.
The neck of the sac increases in the first year or two after grafting.

and barbs,[14] sutures, or staples will be essential. Alternatively, some form of stent-graft that will allow the whole device to expand with an expanding neck may become available.

Of more concern is the number of devices that have started to fail structurally.[15] Many devices are a composite structure of thin graft material and a metal frame. Not surprisingly perhaps, sutures are breaking, and where the metal rubs against the material during cardiac cycles, it is tearing. At least three commercially available grafts have had one of these problems, and when the device fails, so-called type 3 leaks occur with a high chance of rupture. In addition, problems with leakage and dislocation have been seen to occur in the area where the contralateral limb is inserted into the main body of the graft as a separate module. Most commercially available grafts are of a modular design (Fig 3).

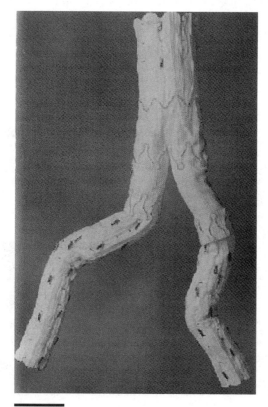

FIGURE 3.
A modular graft.

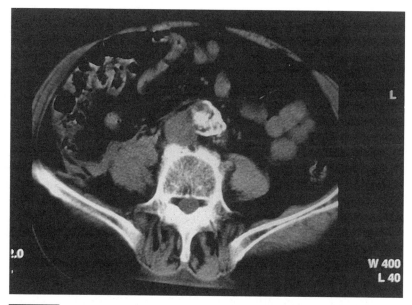

FIGURE 4.
Heavy calcification is a contraindication to endovascular repair.

Lastly, longitudinal shrinkage[8] of the aneurysm sac also occurs with time, leading to dislocation of the stent limbs into the sac with leakage. One problem with this type of damage (type 3 leaks) is that the wall of the aneurysm itself appears to diminish in strength once secure fixation has been obtained. If the graft then leaks because of a structural defect, rupture can occur very rapidly, with a mortality rate of approximately 80%.

When the treatment of patients by endovascular repair first began, a number of patients with unsuitable anatomy such as excessive angulation of the neck were treated. We now know that patients with severe angulation of the neck (>60°), those with heavy calcification (Fig 4) and tortuosity, and those who have poor renal function have a higher mortality rate after endovascular repair, and such patients should probably not be treated.

Currently, the usual upper maximum neck size to be treated is 3 cm. One could argue that this is on the verge of being an aneurysm, and it may be that these patients will be shown to do worse in the long term, although these data are not yet available. Some groups treat patients with necks larger than this. We have to decide which patients should and should not be treated by endovascular methods and recognize that not all of them are suitable candidates for this method of treatment.

ENDOLEAKS

The possibility of leakage occurring from any point where the stent-graft is pressed against the artery remains a problem. If a leak occurs, then clearly the aneurysm sac will remain pressurized and be in danger of rupture. Different types of leakage (endoleak) occur and are classified as follows:

- Type 1 endoleaks suggest that there is leakage from the stent at the top or bottom of the graft as a primary event caused by insecure lodging of the device. These leaks are potentially lethal and must be sealed as soon as possible (Fig 5).
- Type 2 leaks are thought to be caused by back bleeding from the lumbar arteries into the sac, and their importance remains unclear.
- Type 3 leaks are caused by graft disruption. They are associated with a high mortality rate and are very dangerous.
- Type 4 leaks are defined as leakage through thin graft material; their significance is uncertain.

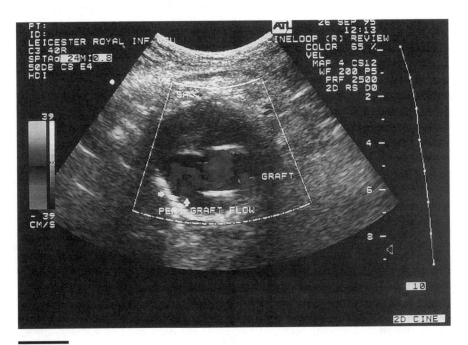

FIGURE 5.
A type 1 endoleak shown by duplex examination.

According to the RETA database,[7] the overall rate of complications was 25% at 30 days, with the endoleak rate being lower in smaller aneurysms than in larger ones and varying between 2% and 10%. A higher endoleak rate, including the type 2 variety, can occur in as many as 18% of patients. These leaks are potentially important, particularly if they cannot be stopped, and the patient may need eventual conversion to open repair. When open repair is needed, the mortality rate is approximately 24%.[8] Endoleaks can probably be prevented or reduced in number by better case selection. We now know that patients with severely angulated necks, those with calcification, and those with thrombus present in the neck of the sac probably should not be treated by endovascular repair. The presence of thrombus acting as an occluding agent between the stent-graft and the neck does not necessarily guarantee that the situation will remain stable in the longer term, because the clot will probably lyse and allow a leak to occur. Bell-shaped necks are also probably unstable, and the graft is more likely to dislocate into the sac.

In regard to type 2 endoleaks, some authors recommend occlusion by embolization of these branches before grafting, but they are in the minority. Plugging the branches with coils before surgery can lead to increased distal embolization, and the branches are often very hard to find. Another technique is to pack the sac with material such as foam to occlude the sac and the vessels. When this technique is used, fewer leaks of this type have been reported to occur. It remains to be seen whether this is the case.

FOLLOW-UP

Most authors now agree that mandatory follow-up, probably at 6-month intervals for life, is necessary for patients who have had an endovascular repair of an aneurysm. Lifetime follow-up is necessary because of the factors already mentioned, such as the tendency for the neck to increase in size and the possibility that the device may dislocate, producing a type 1 endoleak. Disruption of the stent-graft can also obviously occur, making regular assessment essential. Regular follow up inevitably places a strain on the patient who has been treated by an endograft and can lead to stress, particularly because graft failure cannot be forecast. Surveillance includes possible repetitive exposure to ionizing radiation when CT scanning is used. Therefore, duplex scanning with or without contrast is the favored method of examining such patients but is very operator dependent.

No one is really certain how to assess whether the treatment has been successful, but most authors would agree that a shrinking sac is a good indicator that success has been achieved. However, if graft failure occurs in the presence of a shrinking sac, then rupture associated with a high mortality rate is still possible. The clinical significance of a sac that stays the same size is unclear, but it may still indicate that there is a high tension present in the sac.[16] This potential high pressure has been referred to as "endotension," and attempts are being made to find a way of measuring the pressure in the sac in the long term to give an indication of potential leakage. One way of doing this might be to introduce an implantable pressure-measuring device into the sac.

If the sac increases in size, some form of further treatment is mandatory. If an endoleak is present, it should be treated by various endovascular techniques such as inserting coils or further stents. However, if the problem continues, then the patient must be converted to open repair even with the attendant high mortality rate. Because of the uncertainties of knowing exactly what constitutes an effective repair, increasingly sophisticated measurements of the sac size are being made, and volume is now a popular way of trying to assess whether the sac is shrinking.

FURTHER INTERVENTIONS

As one can gather from the above discussion, endoleaks occurring at the rate of about 11% per year are a serious problem. When they occur, attempts have to be made to find out where they are coming from and deal with them. Type 1 endoleaks, if they cannot be stopped by further stenting, have to be converted to open repair; otherwise, rupture will occur. The significance of type 2 endoleaks remains uncertain because it is not known whether they are dangerous. Type 3 endoleaks are the most dangerous, and if they occur, the patient has to be converted immediately or a further stent-graft has to be inserted. An additional problem that occurs mainly with unsupported grafts is occlusion of the contralateral limb, which can occur in as many as 10% of patients. The graft usually can be unblocked by thrombolysis and a wall stent can then be inserted, but sometimes a crossover graft must be put in place to allow the circulation to the leg to continue. If an endoleak at the distal end of the graft persists, it may be necessary to insert an extension into that limb, which may occlude the internal iliac artery. This procedure, if performed on both sides, can cause buttock claudication in as many as 20% of the patients so treated. If the internal iliac arteries are blocked acutely, ischemic colitis or even colonic perforation can occur.

All of these problems lead to uncertainty and impinge on the patient's quality of life. Therefore, a trade-off in terms of short-term gain and long-term loss is something that must be considered.

COST

At present, the average cost of these devices in Europe is approximately $6000, which is an additional item on top of the cost of aneurysm surgery. Most health authorities and private insurance companies will not pay for these devices because they still regard the procedure as experimental and the cost of overall treatment too high. It may be that these costs can be offset by the reduced need for intensive care facilities. However, the savings are more than offset by the need for lifelong follow-up and the complications that require further intervention by stents, coils, or operative procedures. Perhaps in the future, better methods of fixing the graft to the aortic wall will be found that will not necessitate such a long follow-up. This remains to be seen.

Currently, a trial in the United Kingdom has been started called the EVAR Trial (Fig 6). Patients are divided into two groups, EVAR I and EVAR II. In EVAR I, patients who are fit and who are anatomically suitable for endovascular procedures are randomly assigned to receive either open repair or endovascular repair, with appropriate informed consent. It is intended to recruit 800 patients to this trial. The group, EVAR II, aims to compare stenting with best medical treatment in unfit patients. This trial will be of great interest to determine whether stenting is necessary in such patients or confers any benefit. It may be that other disease processes lead to death long before the aneurysm causes a problem. This trial will

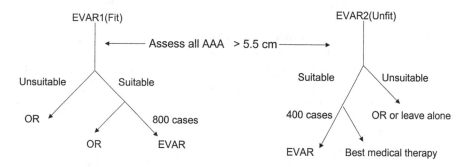

FIGURE 6.
The UK Endovascular *(EVAR)* Versus Open Repair *(OR)* Trial. Five-year follow-up. Each of 5 devices separately tracked. *Abbreviation: AAA,* Abdominal aortic aneurysm.

take at least 5 years to complete and is tracking individual devices in the process. It is not possible to treat a patient by endovascular means in the United Kingdom except in this trial in which costs are fully met. Outside the trial, funds have to be found privately if an endovascular device is inserted. This remains a problem in many European countries.

OVERALL COMMENTS

There is no doubt that stenting of abdominal aortic aneurysms is here to stay. The results, particularly in the grafts that are used to treat small aneurysm of less than 5.5 cm, are very good. However, the small aneurysm trial in the United Kingdom has shown clearly that there is no need, or indication, to treat such lesions because the mortality rate is less than 1% per year if they are left alone. If fit patients are treated, the mortality rate is very low, approximately 1% to 2%, and approximately 6% to 10% for unfit patients. So far, the grafts appear to work, sealing off the aneurysm and leading to a rapid postoperative recovery and good short-term results. The main problem with these grafts remains the need for long-term follow up and the liability of the graft to fatigue and failure, with a high mortality rate. For these reasons, endografts should probably not be used in fit patients except in a randomized trial setting. As for unfit patients, a case can be made for them to be used, although we do not know yet whether the disease process making them unfit will lead to their death long before the aneurysm ruptures. The jury is out, and data will hopefully be provided by the UK trial to allow a verdict. In spite of this, many clinicians are pressing ahead using ever more complicated grafts that will allow branches to be placed in aneurysms above the infrarenal aorta.[17] In addition, success has been achieved in treating ruptured aneurysms.[18] These are two areas in which the technology may well be better placed to succeed. It will be difficult to prove that a device and technique are better than the existing one, which has a mortality rate of 2% to 3% and provides good long-term durability. This is not the case with suprarenal or ruptured aneurysms. I suspect that endovascular repair will be shown to be particularly useful in these areas.

In Europe, we are able to implant almost any graft available because we do not have an organization similar to the Food and Drug Administration. The UK trial currently allows five devices to be implanted and reimbursed. These are the Talent, Ancure, Zenith, AneuRx, and Excluder devices. Each will be tracked separately in the trial.

REFERENCES

1. Fowkes FGR, Macintyre CCA, Ruckley CV: Increasing incidence of aortic aneurysms in England and Wales. *BMJ* 33:298-300, 1989.
2. Johnson KW: Nonruptured abdominal aortic aneurysm: Six year follow up results from the Multicentre Prospective Canadian Aneurysm Study. *J Vasc Surg* 20:163-170, 1994.
3. Zarins CK, Harris EJ Jr: Operative repair for aortic aneurysms: The gold standard. *J Endovasc Surg* 4:232-241, 1999.
4. Volodos NL, Karpovich IP, Shekhanin VE, et al: A case of distant transfemoral endoprosthesis of the thoracic artery using a self-fixing synthetic prosthesis in traumatic aneurysm. *Grud Khirurgiia* 6:84-86, 1988.
5. Parodi JC, Palmaz JC, Barrie HD: Transfemoral, intraluminal graft implantation for abdominal aortic aneurysm. *Ann Vasc Surg* 5:491-499, 1991.
6. The UK Small Aneurysm Trial Participants: Mortality results for randomised controlled trial of early elective surgery or ultrasonographic surveillance for small abdominal aortic aneurysms. *Lancet* 352:1656-1660, 1998.
7. Thomas SM, Gaines PA, Beard JD: Short term (30 day) outcome of endovascular treatment of abdominal aortic aneurysm: Results from the prospective registry of endovascular treatment of abdominal aortic aneurysms (RETA). *Eur J Vasc Endovasc Surg* 21:57-64, 2001.
8. Harris P, Vallaghaneri SR, Desgranges P, et al: Incidence and risk factors of late rupture conversion and death after endovascular repair of infrarenal aortic aneurysms: The Eurostar Experience. *J Vasc Surg* 2:739-749, 2000.
9. Treharne GD, Thompson MM, Bell PRF, et al: Physiological comparison of open and endovascular aneurysm repair. *Br J Surg* 86:760-764, 1999.
10. Thompson MM, Nasim A, Sayvers RD, et al: Oxygen free radical and cytokine generation during endovascular and conventional aneurysm repair. *Eur J Vasc Endovasc Surg* 12:70-75, 1996.
11. Syk I, Brunkwall J, Ivancev K, et al: Postoperative fever, bowel ischaemia and cytokine response to abdominal aortic aneurysm repair: A comparison between open and endovascular surgery. *Eur J Vasc Endovasc Surg* 15:398-405, 1998.
12. Malina M, Lindblath B, Ivancev K: Poor stent graft incorporation in human aortas. *J Endovasc Surg* 5:1S-19S, 1998.
13. Weir JJ, De Nie AJ, Blankenstein JD: Dilatation of the proximal neck of infrarenal aortic aneurysms after endovascular AAA repair. *J Vasc Endovasc Surg* 19:197-201, 2000.
14. Jacobowitz GR, Lee AM, Riles TJ: Immediate and late explantation of endovascular aortic grafts: The endovascular technologies experience. *J Vasc Surg* 29:309-317, 1999.
15. Rieppe G, Heilberger T, Unscheid T, et al: Frame dislocation of body middle rings in endovascular stent tube grafts. *Eur J Vasc Endovasc Surg* 17:28-34, 1998.

16. Rhee RY, Eskandori MK, Zajik AB, et al: Long-term fate of the aneurysm sac after endoluminal exclusion of abdominal aortic aneurysms. *J Vasc Surg* 32:689-696, 2000.

17. Chuter TAM, Gordon RI, Reilly LM, et al: An endovascular system for thoracoabdominal aortic aneurysm repair. *J Endovasc Ther* 8:25-34, 2001.

18. Eith FJ, Ohki T: Newer developments in endovascular graft treatment for aortic and aortoiliac aneurysms. *J Cardiovasc Surg* 41:869-870, 2000.

CHAPTER 4

Evaluation of Aortic Stent Grafting: The Australian Experience

Robert A. Fitridge, MS, FRACS
Senior Lecturer in Vascular Surgery, University of Adelaide, and
Consultant Vascular Surgeon and Head of Vascular Unit, The Queen
Elizabeth Hospital, Adelaide, Australia

After the initial report of placement of an endoluminal stent graft (ELG) for repair of an abdominal aortic aneurysm (AAA) by Parodi[1] in 1991, two Australian groups began working on the application of this technique. The Royal Prince Alfred Hospital (RPAH, Sydney) group, led by May and White, and the Perth group of Lawrence-Brown and Hartley have made many major contributions to the rapid evolution of this technique. Their work has given impetus to the adoption of ELG repair of aneurysms in Australia. These two groups have taken different approaches to the development of the ELG.

The Sydney group performed their first ELG repair in 1992 and have used most of the available stent-graft systems. In addition, they developed a balloon-expandable graft system (the White-Yu device) that they have used extensively. To their credit, this group has carefully studied and reported their early and medium-term results. Their 30-day mortality rate has been approximately 3% to 5%, and they have reported immediate successful aneurysm exclusion in up to 82% of cases, with best results obtained with bifurcated graft systems.[2]

Other contributions of the Sydney group have also included a comparison between first- and second-generation grafts,[3,4] a description of endovascular techniques for dealing with failed exclusion of the aneurysm sac, and open methods used when graft failure has required conversion to open repair.[5] The complications and procedural difficulties that they have encountered have been clearly documented, which has been of great benefit to surgeons commencing ELG repair.

The Perth group first deployed a stent graft in 1993. A small number of tube grafts were used initially. However, since 1994, almost all cases have been performed with the bifurcated graft system that they developed, now called the Zenith graft or H&LB Endograft (Cook Australia, Brisbane, Australia).

Between 1994 and 1998, 238 patients underwent treatment with the Zenith bifurcated graft in Perth. Primary aneurysm exclusion was achieved in 87% of cases, and secondary exclusion was achieved in 94% of cases. Type 1 endoleaks were found in 16% of patients during the follow-up period, of which the majority were sealed with a secondary procedure.[6]

It is a tribute to the designers of this system that it has been proved to be a robust and reliable system that has required minimal modifications since it was first introduced. This graft has been adopted as the graft of choice by the majority of Australian vascular surgeons.

MAJOR ISSUES IN ENDOLUMINAL AAA REPAIR
PATIENT SELECTION CRITERIA

Suitability for ELG repair depends on careful evaluation of the patient and aneurysm morphology. Assessment of aneurysm morphology has been greatly enhanced by the availability of spiral computed tomography angiography (CTA), particularly multislice CTA. This has allowed surgeons and radiologists to assess and plan ELG repair of aneurysms without the need for calibrated catheter angiography. Many Australian groups still routinely perform preoperative angiograms on all patients.

Although there is variation in selection criteria among Australian vascular surgeons, the following criteria are recommended for appropriate utilization of the Zenith graft, the most widely used system in Australia:

1. A proximal neck length of 2 cm (although many surgeons would consider 1.5 cm to be an adequate neck, particularly if using suprarenal fixation). With moderate angulation (between 20° and 45°), a longer (approximately 2.5 cm) neck is required, and severe angulation (>45°) is considered a contraindication.
2. A broad (>2.8 cm) or funnel-shaped neck is an exclusion criterion, as is the presence of a laminated thrombus in the neck. This finding has been more readily apparent with advances in

imaging and is now one of the most frequent contraindications to ELG repair in many surgeons' practices.

3. An iliac artery caliber of less than 7 mm, an iliac artery angulation relative to the axis of the aorta of greater than 60°, and heavily calcified iliac arteries with associated angulation generally exclude aneurysms from this technique. However, the amount of calcification and tortuosity in iliac vessels that is consistent with successful graft deployment is one area in which the surgeon's experience with particular graft types is critical.

4. Unilateral iliac aneurysms with or without a concomitant aortic aneurysm can be excluded, occasionally requiring embolization of the internal iliac artery if the aneurysm extends to within 1.5 cm of the iliac bifurcation. ELG repair can also be performed in cases of bilateral common iliac aneurysms if an adequate distal common iliac "landing zone" is present on at least one side. Maintaining patency of one internal iliac artery is essential.

ENDOLEAK

The term "endoleak" was first proposed in 1996 by White et al[7] from the RPAH group to describe the extravasation of contrast outside the stent graft but within the aneurysm sac (ie, a failure to completely exclude the aneurysm sac from the circulation). This group introduced a classification system based on the site of origin of the endoleak.[8] Clearly defining endoleaks is important because of their contrasting prognosis and management. Early type 1 (proximal or distal graft fixation point) endoleaks are often related to poor case selection, incorrect graft sizing, or deployment problems. If not corrected, early and late type 1 endoleaks result in aneurysm sac expansion, and aneurysm rupture is likely to occur.

Type 2 endoleaks are generally caused by patent lumbar arteries or a patent inferior mesenteric artery backfilling the sac. They are relatively common and are generally associated with maintenance of aneurysm size rather than a decrease in sac size.[9] Many of these endoleaks will thrombose spontaneously with time.

The long-term effects of type 2 endoleaks are unclear, but currently, regular imaging (every 6 months) of the endoleak and close surveillance of aneurysm size are recommended. There appears to be a wide variation in the incidence of type 2 endoleaks after ELG. The more sophisticated the imaging modalities used intra-operatively and at follow-up, the higher the incidence of detection of type 2 endoleaks.

Further modification of endoleak classification has been proposed to include type 3 (defect in the graft fabric, inadequate seal or separation of modular components) and type 4 (porosity of graft fabric).[10]

An interesting recent study from the Perth group[6] examined the relationship between the incidence of type 1 endoleaks after ELG repair and adherence to aneurysm morphology selection guidelines. More than 60% of cases were found to deviate from selection guidelines on one or more parameters, and in these patients, a fourfold increase in type 1 endoleaks was found. The presence of more than one exclusion criterion greatly increased the incidence of endoleak.

ENDOTENSION

"Endotension" is a term developed to describe the finding of aneurysm sac expansion after ELG repair without an endoleak being demonstrated. The term was first used in 1999 by Gilling-Smith et al[11] and White et al.[12] Endotension appears likely to be caused by transmission of pressure into the aneurysm sac via thrombus present at fixation points, or transmission of pressure through the graft material. This diagnosis requires exclusion of endoleak via standard, high-definition imaging techniques. However, low-flow endoleak cannot be excluded as the etiology of this problem.

SURVEILLANCE

After implantation of an ELG, a spiral CTA is obtained within 10 days of the procedure. In the absence of endoleak, routine surveillance comprises spiral CTA every 6 months for 1 year, then annually thereafter, assuming the aneurysm sac does not increase in size. Some groups with special expertise have developed the duplex scan as their primary imaging modality for surveillance.

The presence of a type 2 endoleak requires ongoing surveillance every 6 months. Type 1 endoleaks, aneurysm sac expansion, or both, require angiography. Intervention is required to prevent aneurysm rupture.

COST-EFFECTIVENESS OF ELG REPAIR IN AUSTRALIA

A recent Australian study[13] of two well-matched groups showed that the cost of preoperative imaging, in-hospital care, early readmission, and follow-up costs were 50% greater in the ELG patients compared with those undergoing open repair. The costs of the graft, surveillance costs, and the requirement for reintervention outweighed the savings of a shorter hospital stay and a reduced intensive therapy unit stay in Australian practice.

DURABILITY

Perhaps the most important issue facing ELG is the durability of this procedure. The rate of reintervention in the EUROSTAR registry of more than 1000 patients is 18% at a mean of 14 months. At 3 years, 33% of patients had undergone a variety of secondary interventional procedures.[14] The Sydney group has reported a 3-year graft success probability of 82%.[3] Similarly, Holzenbein et al[15] performed additional interventions in 27% of their ELG cases at a mean of 18 months.

Proximal neck dilatation in patients after ELG repair is a major issue for this technique. Makaroun et al[16] found that 21% of patients had developed a mean proximal neck dilatation of 4.8 mm at 2 years after ELG placement. White et al[17] demonstrated an average aortic dilatation of 0.9 mm at the level of the renal arteries in the first year, which appeared to progress slowly. These findings suggest that there is a risk that gradual proximal neck dilatation may occur after ELG repair, and if this results in the aortic neck dilating beyond the diameter of the self-expanding graft (usually oversized 2-4 mm), proximal type 1 endoleaks are likely to develop.

ZENITH GRAFT

The Zenith graft is a fully supported bifurcated graft system that uses self-expanding Z stents. The graft material is woven Dacron. An uncovered proximal Gianturco Z stent with attachment hooks is incorporated into the graft, so that in all cases, suprarenal fixation is used.[18]

Initially, all grafts were custom-made; however, the "Trifab" graft system (Cook Australia) has recently been developed (Fig 1). This modular graft system is essentially the same as the custom-made graft, except that an extension limb on both sides is required. This allows the graft system to be obtained "off the shelf" without necessitating a delay for customized graft construction.

Aneurysms with relatively short proximal necks (<1.5 cm) and juxtarenal aneurysms are unsuitable for ELG repair with standard graft systems. An approach to overcome this problem has been developed by the Perth group.[19] The fenestrated graft is designed to obtain proximal fixation in the suprarenal or supraceliac aorta. Fenestrations are cut into the proximal body of the graft to allow graft extensions to be passed into targeted renal vessels, mesenteric vessels, or both.

The fenestrations lie between two Dacron-covered Z stents. Radiopaque markers allow accurate positioning of the target vessel

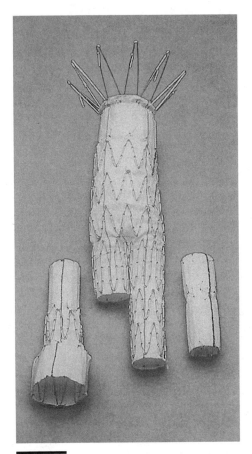

FIGURE 1.
Trifab graft (Cook Australia).

ostium. A trigger wire, which is incorporated into the standard Perth graft, ensures incomplete graft expansion until precise graft positioning has been obtained (Figs 2 and 3).

The initial report described stent-graft placement in an experimental model.[19] Since this time, a number of grafts have been deployed in patients.[20] This technically challenging modification requires detailed preoperative spiral CTA imaging as well as precise intraoperative graft positioning. Open resection of juxtarenal or short-necked infrarenal aneurysms is considered relatively straightforward by most experienced vascular surgeons. The short- and medium-term results of this complex and challenging endovascular treatment are awaited with interest.

GOVERNMENT REGULATION OF ELG REPAIR IN AUSTRALIA

The Commonwealth Minister for Health created the Medicare Services Advisory Committee (MSAC) in 1998 to assess the safety, efficacy, and cost-effectiveness of new techniques and technologies being introduced into clinical practice. ELG repair of AAA was one of these procedures. This review essentially concluded that the ELG repair of AAA appears to be effective in the short term, but that there were insufficient data to assess the long-term safety and durability of the procedure. There was criticism of the lack of randomized controlled trial evidence to support the ELG technique.[21]

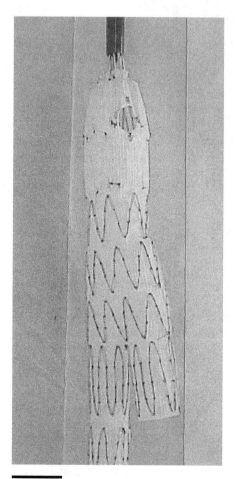

FIGURE 2.
Fenestrated Zenith graft (Cook Australia).

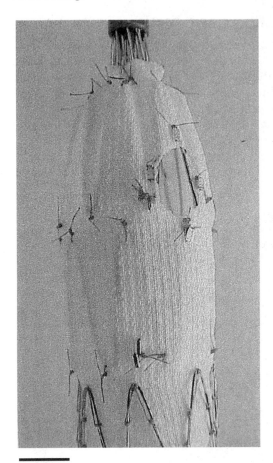

FIGURE 3.
Detail of fenestration—Zenith graft (Cook Australia).

AUSTRALIAN SAFETY AND EFFICACY REGISTER OF NEW INTERVENTIONAL PROCEDURES–SURGICAL

The Australian Safety and Efficacy Register of New Interventional Procedures–Surgical (ASERNIP-S) arose under the auspices of the Royal Australasian College of Surgeons and is funded by the Australian Government. The aim of this project is to assess the safety and efficacy of new surgical procedures before their use in routine clinical practice.

After release of the MSAC Review of ELG for AAA, the Australian Government funded ASERNIP-S to develop and manage a national database to evaluate endoluminal and open aortic aneurysm repair. Data sets were designed for (1) patient demographics and procedural information; (2) discharge/30-day follow-up; (3) 6-month follow-up; (4) 12-month follow-up; and (5) thereafter annual review.

Clearly, one of the major issues for endoluminal grafting is the long-term durability of the procedure, and thus, follow-up data of the patients whose initial results have been submitted to ASERNIP-S will be closely monitored over the medium to long term.

Data have been collected since November 1999 on a voluntary basis. Analysis has been performed on the first 12 months of data collection. A total of 829 cases were reported to ASERNIP-S during the first year. This included 474 patients undergoing ELG and 355 undergoing open AAA repair.

RESULTS OF ASERNIP-S DATABASE

After contact with vascular surgeons via the Royal Australasian College of Surgeons, the Commonwealth Department of Health, and stent manufacturers, ASERNIP-S found that 104 of the 150 vascular surgeons in Australia are currently performing ELG repair. A total of 132 surgeons reported performing open AAA repair. During the period of data collection, 91 surgeons have submitted ELG cases.[22]

Comorbidities in both open and ELG groups were evenly matched. In the ELG data set, just over 50% of patients were aged 74 years or younger, and 53% of aneurysms were 5.5 cm or less in diameter (approximately 17% of aneurysms were 4.9 cm or less in diameter).

Site of ELG Procedure

A majority of surgeons in Australia have decided that because of the importance of high-quality imaging, ELG repair should be performed in the angiography suite or dedicated endovascular suites. Less than one third of procedures were undertaken in the operating room with mobile image intensification. General anesthesia has been used in more than 70% of ELG cases. Just under 30% of cases were performed with patients under epidural, spinal, or local anesthesia. Open access of the femoral artery has been used in approximately 95% of cases for the body of the graft and in more than 80% of cases for the contralateral limb.

Graft Types

Currently, seven grafts are being used in Australia; however, the Zenith (Cook Australia) graft has been inserted in more than 85%

of cases during the review period. Approximately 90% of all grafts in the submitted data have been of the aorto-bi-iliac bifurcated configuration.

Morbidity and Mortality

The 30-day mortality rate was less than 3% in both ELG and open groups. Vascular and graft-related complications occurred at the time of the procedure in 15% of cases in both groups (Tables 1 and 2). A further 7% of patients who had ELG procedures developed graft complications before discharge, all of which required further intervention.

The majority of complications associated with ELG procedures relate to access site complications and problems with graft seal and deployment. The incidence of type 1 and type 2 endoleaks (3% and 5%, respectively) is comparatively low in this reported series. Postoperative systemic (mainly cardiorespiratory) complications other than pyrexia are less common in the ELG group than in the open group (40% vs 70% after open repair).

Patient admission to the intensive care unit occurred in 30% of ELG cases and 67% of open cases. The mean length of hospital admission was 7.3 days for ELG repair versus 14.6 days in the open group. Transfused blood products within 24 hours were reported in 9% of ELG patients versus 32% of patients who had open repairs.

Follow-up

Perhaps the most valuable role of this database administered by ASERNIP-S will prove to be in tracking the medium- to long-term outcomes of patients in the ASERNIP-S database. Contact is made with surgeons when follow-up data are due, and this study will provide useful long-term durability data.

TABLE 1.
Vascular and Graft Complications at Time of ELG Procedure

Complication	Proportion (N = 474)
Failed access/access vessel complications	2.7%
Failed/misplaced deployment	1.2%
Imperfect seal	4.4%
Graft twist/occlusion	2.1%
Other	4.8%
Total	15.2%

Abbreviation: ELG, Endoluminal stent graft.

TABLE 2.
Complications at Time of Open AAA Repair

Complication	Proportion
Myocardial infarction	2.9%
Arrhythmia	3.2%
Ischemic leg	1.2%
Ischemic gut	0.6%
Other	7.0%
Total	14.9%

Abbreviation: AAA, Abdominal aortic aneurysm.

ACKNOWLEDGMENTS

The author acknowledges the role of the Medicare Services Advisory Committee of the Commonwealth Department of Health in commissioning the ASERNIP-S database. This review of contemporary Australian experience would not have been possible without kind access to the ASERNIP-S data and the enthusiastic assistance of Professor G. Maddern (Surgical Director of ASERNIP-S) and Dr W. Babidge and M. Boult (Researchers, ASERNIP-S).

REFERENCES

1. Parodi JC: Transfemoral intraluminal graft implantation for abdominal aortic aneurysms. *Ann Vasc Surg* 6:491-499, 1991.
2. May J, White GH, Yu W, et al: Importance of graft configuration in outcome of endoluminal aortic aneurysm repair: A 5-year analysis by life table method. *Eur J Vasc Endovasc Surg* 15:406-411, 1998.
3. May J, White GH, Harris JP: Techniques for surgical conversion of aortic endoprosthesis. *Eur J Vasc Endovasc Surg* 18:284-289, 1999.
4. May J, White GH, Waugh R, et al: Comparison of first- and second-generation prostheses for endoluminal repair of abdominal aortic aneurysms: A 6-year study with life table analysis. *J Vasc Surg* 32:124-129, 2000.
5. May J, White GH, Yu W, et al: Endoluminal grafting of abdominal aortic aneurysms: Causes and failure and their prevention. *J Endovasc Surg* 1:44-52, 1994.
6. Stanley BM, Semmens JB, Mai Q, et al: Evaluation of patient selection guidelines for endoluminal grafting of aneurysm of the abdominal aorta with the Zenith graft: The Australian experience. *J Endovas Ther*, in press.
7. White GH, Yu W, May J: Endoleak: A proposed new terminology to describe incomplete aneurysm exclusion by an endoluminal graft (letter). *J Endovasc Surg* 3:124-125, 1996.
8. White GH, Yu W, May J, et al: Endoleak as a complication of en-

doluminal grafting of abdominal aortic aneurysms: Classification, incidence, diagnosis and management. *J Endovasc Surg* 4:152-168, 1997.

9. Wolf YG, Hill BB, Rubin GD, et al: Rate of change in abdominal aortic aneurysm diameter after endovascular repair. *J Vasc Surg* 32:108-115, 2000.

10. White GH, May J, Waugh RC, et al: Type III and Type IV endoleak: Toward a complete definition of blood flow in the sac after endoluminal AAA repair. *J Endovasc Surg* 5:305-309, 1998.

11. Gilling-Smith G, Brennan J, Harris P, et al: Endotension after endovascular aneurysm repair: Definition, classification and strategies for surveillance and intervention. *J Endovasc Surg* 6:305-307, 1999.

12. White GH, May J, Petrasek P: Endotension: An explanation for continued AAA growth after successful endoluminal repair. *J Endovasc Surg* 6:308-315, 1999.

13. Birch SE, Stary DR, Scott AR: Cost of endovascular versus open surgical repair of abdominal aortic aneurysms. *Aust N Z J Surg* 70:660-666, 2000.

14. Leheij RJF, Buth J, Harris PL, et al: Need for secondary interventions after endovascular repair of abdominal aortic aneurysms. Intermediate-term follow-up results of a European collaborative registry (EUROSTAR). *Br J Surg* 87:1666-1673, 2000.

15. Holzenbein TJ, Kretschmer G, Thurnher S, et al: Midterm durability of abdominal aortic aneurysm endograft repair: A word of caution. *J Vasc Surg* 33:S46-S54, 2001.

16. Makaroun MS, and the Endovascular Technologies Investigators: Is proximal aortic neck dilatation after endovascular aneurysm exclusion a cause for concern? *J Vasc Surg* 33:S39-S45, 2001.

17. White RA, Donayre CE, Walot I, et al: Computed tomography assessment of abdominal aortic aneurysm morphology after endograft exclusion. *J Vasc Surg* 33:S1-S10, 2001.

18. Van Schie GP, Sieunatine K, Lawrence-Brown MMD, et al: The Perth bifurcated endovascular graft for infrarenal aortic aneurysms. *Semin Interv Radiol* 15:63-69, 1998.

19. Browne TF, Hartley D, Purchas S, et al: A fenestrated covered suprarenal aortic stent. *Eur J Vasc Endovasc Surg* 18:445-449, 1999.

20. Anderson JL, Berce M, Hartley DE: Endoluminal aortic grafting with renal and superior mesenteric artery incorporation by graft fenestration. *J Endovasc Ther* 8:3-15, 2001.

21. Medicare Services Advisory Committee (MSAC): *Endoluminal Grafting for Abdominal Aortic Aneurysm. Final Assessment Report.* Canberra, Australia, Commonwealth Department of Health and Aged Care, 1999, pp 1-23.

22. Australian Safety and Efficacy Register of New Interventional Procedures–Surgical (ASERNIP-S): *Audit of Endoluminal and Open Repair of Abdominal Aortic Aneurysms. First Annual Report to the Commonwealth Department of Health and Aged Care.* Adelaide, Australia, ASERNIP-S, 2001, pp 1-109.

C HAPTER 5

Management of the Various Types of Endoleaks*

Takao Ohki, MD
Associate Professor of Surgery, Albert Einstein College of Medicine, and
Chief, Endovascular Program, Montefiore Medical Center, New York, NY

Frank J. Veith, MD
Professor of Surgery, Albert Einstein College of Medicine, and Chief,
Vascular Surgery, Montefiore Medical Center, New York, NY

Since endovascular aortic aneurysm repair (EVAR) has been proved to be safe and minimally invasive in the short term, it has gained wide acceptance. Its value in patients with large aneurysms that are deemed inoperable because of serious comorbid conditions, hostile abdomens, or both, is apparent. However, its role in the treatment of healthy patients who are good surgical candidates has yet to be determined because of the occurrence of early and late failures. Endoleaks continue to be the most common causes of both early and late failures.[1-8]

An endoleak is defined as perigraft blood flow within the aneurysm sac. Endoleaks have been classified into four types (Fig 1): endoleaks associated with incomplete sealing of proximal and distal fixation sites (type 1 [Figs 2-4]); retrograde flow from collateral branches (type 2 [Figs 5 and 6]); defects in the stent-graft itself or disconnection of the limbs (type 3 [Figs 7 and 8]); and graft porosity (type 4 [Fig 9]).[1-3] An endoleak can be present immediately after surgery (primary) or may develop after initially not being apparent (secondary). This chapter outlines the significance of various endoleaks as well as treatment strategies based on existing evidence.

---

*Supported by grants from the US Public Health Service (HL 02990-05), the James Hilton Manning and Emma Austin Manning Foundation, and the Anna S. Brown Trust.

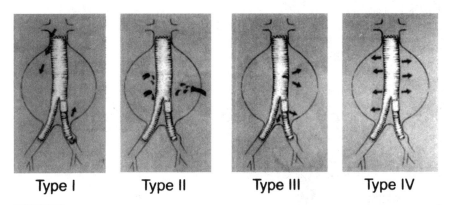

Type I   Type II   Type III   Type IV

FIGURE 1.

Classification of endoleaks. (Courtesy of White GH, May J, Waugh RC, et al: Type III and IV endoleak: Toward a complete definition of blood flow in the sac after endoluminal AAA repair. *J Endovasc Surg* 5:305-309, 1998. Used by permission.)

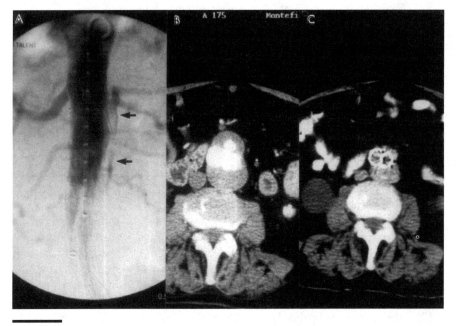

FIGURE 2.

Example of a long and narrow type 1 endoleak successfully treated by inducing thrombosis. **A,** A long, narrow type 1 endoleak *(arrows)* can be seen. **B,** Postoperative CT scan shows a 5.5-cm aneurysm with a type 1 endoleak. **C,** Thrombosis of this endoleak was induced by temporarily terminating chronic anticoagulation therapy. Eighteen months after endovascular repair, the aneurysm has almost completely disappeared.

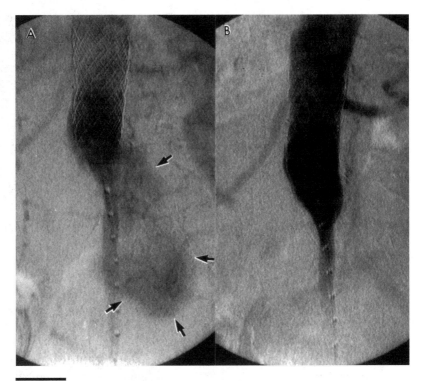

FIGURE 3.
A, A secondary type 1 endoleak with a short, large channel that developed 12 months after initial surgery. *Arrows* denote a type 1 endoleak. **B,** This endoleak was managed by deploying a second endovascular graft (EVG) within the first EVG.

SIGNIFICANCE OF TYPE 1 AND TYPE 3 ENDOLEAKS

There is considerable debate as well as confusion regarding the clinical significance of an endoleak detected on postoperative imaging studies. Some authors have stated that the presence or absence of some endoleaks does not affect the efficacy of the treatment,[9-11] whereas we and others believe that any form of endoleak should be considered as at least a potential treatment failure. In addition, according to the Society for Vascular Surgery/International Society for Cardiovascular Surgery reporting standards, the presence of any endoleak is defined as a treatment failure.[12] Although different opinions regarding the significance of a type 2 endoleak exist, there is an almost universal consensus that type 1 and type 3 endoleaks should be treated if at all possible.

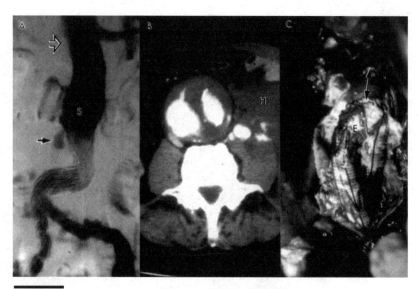

FIGURE 4.
Late failure managed by open conversion. **A,** A secondary type 1 endoleak *(closed arrow)* developed during follow-up. This endoleak was caused by migration of the proximal stent *(S)*. Note the excessive kink of the endovascular graft (EVG) caused by migration. *Open arrow* denotes the location in which the proximal stent was initially deployed. **B,** CT scan reveals an endoleak. In addition, the aneurysm has ruptured and a retroperitoneal hematoma *(H)* can be seen. **C,** Open conversion was performed on an urgent basis. The proximal part of the EVG was excised, and the remainder of the EVG *(E)* was bridged to the proximal neck with a short segment of standard graft *(arrow)*.

SIGNIFICANCE OF A TYPE 2 ENDOLEAK

Intuition tells us that a type 2 endoleak is less harmful when compared with a type 1 or a type 3 endoleak because it has a lower flow and presumably a lower pressure. In fact, the recent report from EUROSTAR has provided some evidence to support this concept.[4] In this report, the significant risk factors for aneurysm growth and subsequent rupture after EVAR were the presence of type 1 and type 3 endoleaks and graft migration. The presence of a type 2 endoleak was not a significant risk factor. Therefore, some authors have termed type 2 as a minor rather than a major endoleak. However, a recent study by Baum et al[13] has shown that systemic pressure is transmitted into the aneurysm sac with type 2 endoleaks. These authors measured intra-aneurysmal sac pressure by placing a needle into the sac via a translumbar approach in patients with various types of endoleaks. Their results clearly showed that all patent endoleaks, including type 2 endoleaks, transmit systemic pressure to the aneurysm sac. In addition, there have been sporadic reports of aneurysm rupture after a type 2 endoleak. Although an aneurysm with a type 2 endoleak that has not grown or shrunk on subsequent CT scans may be treated conservatively, those that enlarge clearly need some form of treatment.

TREATMENT OPTIONS FOR VARIOUS TYPES OF ENDOLEAKS

Various methods for the treatment of endoleaks have been attempted. Options for treating endoleaks include coil embolization (transarterial and translumbar access), the addition of stent-graft cuffs and extensions, laparoscopic ligation of the inferior mesenteric and lumbar arteries, redo endovascular stent-graft repair, and open surgical

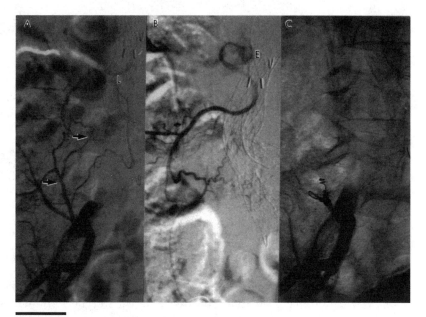

FIGURE 5.
An example of a type 2 endoleak. **A,** Injection of the right hypogastric artery shows the iliolumbar artery *(arrows)* feeding the lumbar artery *(L)* and the endoleak. **B,** Selective injection further denotes the connection between the iliolumbar artery, lumbar artery, and the endoleak *(E).* Note the presence of multiple arteries communicating with the lumbar artery feeding the aneurysm. **C,** Coil embolization of the orifice of the iliolumbar artery was performed. However, because of the presence of multiple communicating arteries, this treatment was not effective and the endoleak persisted.

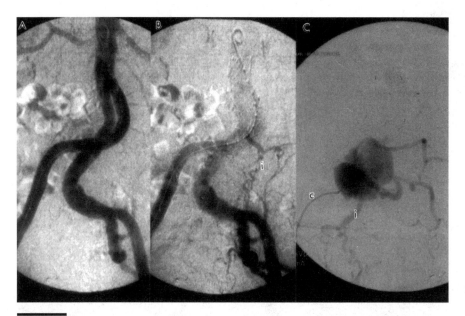

FIGURE 6.
Translumbar access for the diagnosis and treatment of an endoleak. **A,** This patient is 12 months status post endovascular aortic aneurysm repair. At 12 months, the CT scan showed enlargement of the aneurysm as well as the presence of an endoleak. A transfemoral angiogram was initially obtained, since it was felt that the endoleak was type 3. **B,** However, the angiogram revealed a type 2 endoleak arising from the left iliolumbar artery *(i)*. **C,** Translumbar access of the aneurysm revealed the presence of multiple feeding arteries in addition to the iliolumbar artery *(i)* shown on a standard angiogram. Sac pressure was equivalent to systemic blood pressure. Selective coil embolization of each lumbar artery was performed, which resulted in successful outcome. *Abbreviation: c,* translumbar catheter.

repair. A recent article by White and May[14] summarizes these treatment options (Table 1). This strategy stratifies the treatment based on the classification of endoleaks. It assumes that all endoleaks categorized into a particular type are equal (eg, all type 1 endoleaks are equal). However, we believe that even if they are classified as the same type of endoleak, certain differences between these endoleaks may affect the method of treatment.

EXPERIMENTAL RESEARCH DATA TO SUPPORT THE CONCEPT THAT "NOT ALL ENDOLEAKS ARE EQUAL"

We and others have conducted several animal and bench studies to better understand the significance of endoleaks.[15-18]

EX VIVO CIRCULATORY ANEURYSM MODEL

In an ex vivo model,[18] endoleak channels of various lengths were constructed using polytetrafluoroethylene (PTFE) grafts and then attached to an artificial aneurysm sac. These endoleak channels were incorporated within a mock circulation connected to a pulsatile pump. Pressure in the aneurysm sac was recorded distal to each endoleak channel. Subsequently, the endoleak channels were filled with human thrombus to mimic thrombosed or sealed endoleaks, and the pressure measurements were repeated. In the absence of thrombus, the pressure did not change across the endoleak channels, regardless of channel length or diameter. In the presence of organized thrombus, the pressure distal to the endoleak channels was reduced to a degree directly proportional to the length and inversely proportional to the diameter of the endoleak channel (Fig 10).

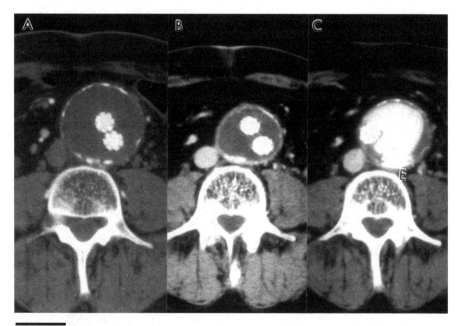

FIGURE 7.

A, CT scan obtained immediately postoperatively shows complete exclusion of the aneurysm with no signs of an endoleak. **B,** Follow-up CT scan obtained 12 months postoperatively revealed shrinkage of the aneurysm. **C,** At 18 months, the junction of the contralateral limb of the bifurcated endovascular graft (EVG) became separated and resulted in a type 3 endoleak and acute enlargement of the sac. Note the distorted left limb of the EVG *(E)*. This endoleak was successfully treated by bridging the separated portion with an extension limb.

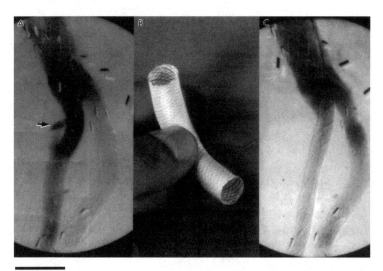

FIGURE 8.

A, An example of a type 3 endoleak *(arrow)* caused by a fabric tear. **B,** Since the endoleak channel was wide and short, it was necessary to cover the orifice rather than perform a coil embolization. A covered stent was used to treat this leak. **C,** A covered stent was successfully deployed across the endoleak channel, which resulted in resolution of the endoleak.

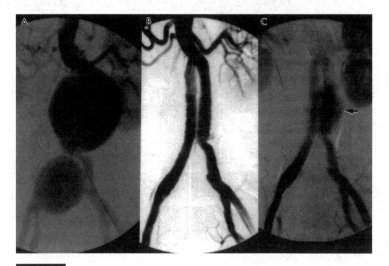

FIGURE 9.

A, A preoperative angiogram shows a complex aneurysm. **B,** Endovascular aortic aneurysm repair was successfully performed after coil embolization of the right hypogastric artery. There are no type 1, 2, or 3 endoleaks. **C,** A type 4 endoleak *(arrow)* can be seen. This type of endoleak will usually resolve spontaneously once the effect of anticoagulation wears off.

TABLE 1.
Proposed Classification of Endoleaks

Endoleak Classification	Alternative Terms	Forms	Therapeutic Alternatives
Type I	Attachment endoleak Perigraft channel Perigraft leak Graft-related endoleak	Proximal graft attachment zone Distal attachment zone Occluder plug region Occluder plug region	Proximal or distal extension or cuff Embolization Secondary endograft Open repair
Type II	Retrograde endoleak Collateral flow Retroleak Non–graft-related endoleak	Patent lumbar artery Patent IMA Patent intercostal artery Others (accessory renal artery, internal iliac, subclavian, etc)	Conservative Coil embolization Laparoscopic clip application Laparoscopic clip application
Type III	Fabric tear Modular disconnection or poor seal	Midgraft fabric tear Contralateral stump disconnection	Secondary endograft Secondary endograft
Type IV	Porosity	Graft wall fabric porosity; suture holes	Conservative
Undefined origin Endotension	Endopressure Pressure leak Pseudoendoleak Type V endoleak	High pressure in sac, but no endoleak detectable Thrombotic seal	Secondary endograft Open repair Others?

Abbreviation: IMA, Inferior mesenteric artery.
(Courtesy of White GH, May J: How should endotension be defined? *J Endovasc Ther* 7:435–438, 2000. Used by permission.)

This ex vivo model suggests that endoleaks with longer channels and smaller diameters would derive greater benefit from adjunctive maneuvers that hasten thrombosis. On the other hand, thrombosis of endoleaks with short and wide channels may not result in substantial pressure reduction within the aneurysm sac.

CHRONIC ANEURYSM PRESSURE MEASUREMENTS IN CANINES

Pressure transducers were implanted in the wall of an experimental aneurysm constructed from PTFE and then implanted in dogs. This model permitted the measurement of pressure within the aneurysm sac on a chronic basis. The aneurysm pressure was measured before and after various endovascular treatments. Initially, different endovascular grafts (EVGs) with different graft materials and different porosities were tested. Although, based on angiogram and CT scan findings, both the low- and the high-porosity grafts were able to achieve complete exclusion, the intra-aneurysmal pressure was reduced only with the use of the low-porosity graft.[15]

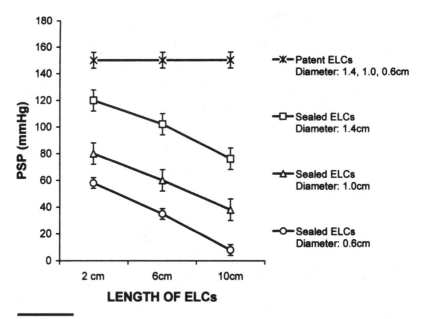

FIGURE 10.
Pressure transmission across patent and thrombosed endoleak channels *(ELCs)* depending on their length and diameter. *Abbreviation: PSP,* Peak systolic pressure. (Courtesy of Mehta M, Ohki T, Veith FJ, et al: All sealed endoleaks are not the same: A treatment strategy based on an ex vivo analysis. *Eur J Vasc Endovasc Surg* 21:541-544, 2001. Used by permission.)

We then investigated the effect of a short, wide endoleak.[16] Low-porosity PTFE EVGs with an artificial hole (diameter, 4 mm) mimicking a type 3 endoleak were deployed to treat an experimental aneurysm. Not surprisingly, the intra-aneurysmal pressure remained at the systemic level. We next investigated the effectiveness of inducing thrombosis by deploying embolization coils into the endoleak. Based on CT scan and angiogram findings, the endoleak channel completely sealed, but the intrasac pressure remained at the systemic level. In both animal studies, angiograms and CT scans failed to detect a treatment failure. Furthermore, inducing thrombosis was not effective for large, short endoleak channels.

These experimental models suggest that when the endoleak has a long and narrow channel, the pressure transmission across the thrombus may be significantly reduced; thus, inducing thrombosis may lead to a successful outcome. On the other hand, endoleak channels with a short and wide diameter require that the hole be covered with graft material to obliterate pressure transmission. These data suggest that it is not the type of endoleak that should dictate treatment strategy. Rather, it should in part be determined based on the length and diameter of the endoleak channel.

We have applied this concept in the treatment of endoleaks in a clinical scenario. In clinical cases, most type 2 endoleaks have a long, narrow channel, whereas most type 1 and type 3 endoleaks have a short, wide channel. However, there are several exceptions. Because some type 1 and type 3 endoleaks may have a short, narrow channel, inducing thrombosis may lead to effective pressure reduction (Fig 11).

TREATMENT STRATEGY

SHORT AND WIDE ENDOLEAK CHANNELS (INCLUDES MOST TYPE 1 AND TYPE 3 ENDOLEAKS)

As described earlier, hastening thrombosis with coils will most likely not be effective, and it will be necessary to either cover the endoleak orifice with a new EVG or convert to a surgical repair (Figs 3, 4, 7, and 8). In most instances, deployment of a second EVG or an extension cuff is possible, but one should not hesitate to convert if an endovascular approach is not possible.

LONG AND NARROW ENDOLEAK CHANNELS

Most type 2 endoleaks will have long, narrow channels and they will, therefore, benefit from inducing thrombosis. Methods for inducing thrombosis include temporarily terminating chronic anticoagulation therapy, coil embolization, or injection of glue. As for the

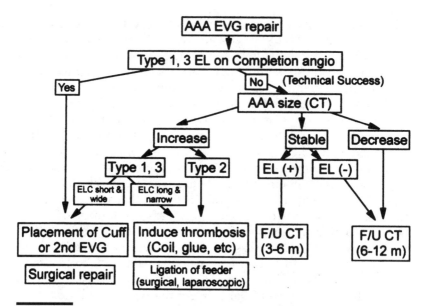

FIGURE 11.
Treatment strategies for various types of endoleaks. *Abbreviations: AAA,* Abdominal aortic aneurysm; *EVG,* endovascular graft; *EL,* endoleak; *CT,* computed tomography; *ELC,* endoleak channel; *F/U,* follow-up.

method of access, either a transarterial or a translumbar approach can be used. Because most type 2 endoleaks have more than one inflow/outflow, it may be difficult to coil embolize all the endoleak channels via a transarterial approach (Fig 5). We therefore currently recommend using a translumbar approach for all type 2 endoleaks (Fig 6). In addition to type 2 endoleaks, some type 1 or type 3 endoleaks have long, narrow channels. These endoleaks can be effectively treated with coil embolization or other methods to hasten thrombosis (Fig 2).

CONCEPT OF ENDOTENSION

We and others have experienced aneurysm growth in the absence of an endoleak. This has been termed "endotension."[14,19] Endotension is defined as pressurization of an aneurysm sac after EVAR without evidence of an endoleak. "Endoleak" applies only when there is demonstrable flow outside the EVG. However, as shown by our animal model, not all sealed endoleaks result in pressure reduction in the aneurysm. When a short, wide endoleak channel undergoes thrombosis, the endoleak will no longer be seen on a CT scan or an angiogram, but the pressure may be transmitted into the sac. Thus, endotension may occur when a short, wide endoleak channel undergoes thrombosis or when an EVG migrates and exposes a large area of aneurysm thrombus to the main aortic blood flow and pressure. There are other causes of endotension, including infection and sweating of the EVG, as well as other mechanisms that are not yet clearly understood. At this time, open surgical conversion is the only effective method to treat this phenomenon, although the outcome of observational treatment remains unknown.

SUMMARY

Based on recent reports regarding the midterm results, it is clear that EVAR is not as durable as open repair and thus may not be a definitive procedure. Therefore, lifelong surveillance is mandatory and is an important part of the overall treatment. Failure to detect a late failure may lead to aneurysm rupture.

Although EVAR may fail secondary to EVG migration or an endoleak, it can usually be treated with another endovascular procedure. Therefore, we do not necessarily consider late failure as a defeat.[6,8] Treatment methods include a variety of endovascular and even laparoscopic techniques, as well as open conversion. The treatment should be based on the type of endoleak and the presence or absence of aneurysm enlargement. Treatment methods should be individualized based on the length and diameter of the endoleak channel.

REFERENCES

1. White GH, May J, Waugh R, et al: Type I and type II endoleaks: A more useful classification for reporting results of endoluminal AAA repair. *J Endovasc Surg* 5:189-193, 1998.
2. Wain RA, Marin ML, Ohki T, et al: Endoleaks after endovascular graft treatment of aortic aneurysms: Classification, risk factors, and outcome. *J Vasc Surg* 27:69-80, 1998.
3. White GH, May J, Waugh RC, et al: Type III and IV endoleak: Toward a complete definition of blood flow in the sac after endoluminal AAA repair. *J Endovasc Surg* 5:305-309, 1998.
4. Peter L, Harris S, Vallabhaneni R, et al: Incidence and risk factors of late rupture, conversion, and death after endovascular repair of infrarenal aortic aneurysms: The EUROSTAR experience. *J Vasc Surg* 32:739-749, 2000.
5. Bush RL, Lumsden AB, Dodson TF, et al: Mid-term results after endovascular repair of the abdominal aortic aneurysm. *J Vasc Surg* 33:70S-76S, 2001.
6. Laheij RJ, Buth J, Harris PL, et al: Need for secondary interventions

after endovascular repair of abdominal aortic aneurysms. Intermediate-term follow-up results of a European collaborative registry
(EUROSTAR). *Br J Surg* 87:1666-1673, 2000.

7. Hölzenbein TJ, Kretschmer G, Thurnher S, et al: Midterm durability
   of abdominal aortic aneurysm endograft repair: A word of caution.
   J Vasc Surg 33:46S-54S, 2001.

8. Ohki T, Veith FJ, Shaw P, et al: Increasing incidence of mid and long-
   term complications after endovascular graft repair of AAAs: A note of
   caution based on an 8-year experience with 212 cases. *Ann Surg*, in
   press.

9. Rhee RY, Eskandari MK, Zajko AB, et al: Long-term fate of the aneurysmal sac after endoluminal exclusion of abdominal aortic aneurysms. *J Vasc Surg* 32:689-696, 2000.

10. Zarins CK, White RA, Moll FL, et al: The AneuRx stent graft: Four-
    year results and worldwide experience 2000. *J Vasc Surg* 33:135S-
    145S, 2001.

11. Resch T, Ivancev K, Lindh M, et al: Persistent collateral perfusion of
    abdominal aortic aneurysm after endovascular repair does not lead to
    progressive change in aneurysm diameter. *J Vasc Surg* 28:242-249,
    1998.

12. Ahn SS, Rutherford RB, Johnston KW, et al: Reporting standards for
    infrarenal endovascular abdominal aortic aneurysm repair. Ad Hoc
    Committee for Standardized Reporting Practices in Vascular Surgery
    of The Society for Vascular Surgery/International Society for
    Cardiovascular Surgery. *J Vasc Surg* 25:405-410, 1997.

13. Baum RA, Carpenter JP, Cope C, et al: Aneurysm sac pressure mea-
    surements after endovascular repair of abdominal aortic aneurysms.
    J Vasc Surg 33:32-41, 2001.

14. White GH, May J: How should endotension be defined? History of a
    concept and evolution of a new term. *J Endovasc Ther* 7:435-438, 2000.

15. Sanchez LA, Faries PL, Marin ML, et al: Chronic intraaneurysmal
    pressure measurement: An experimental method for evaluating the
    effectiveness of endovascular aortic aneurysm exclusion. *J Vasc Surg*
    26:222-230, 1997.

16. Marty B, Sanchez LA, Ohki T, et al: Endoleak after endovascular graft
    repair of experimental aortic aneurysms: Does coil embolization with
    angiographic "seal" lower intraaneurysmal pressure? *J Vasc Surg*
    27:454-462, 1998.

17. Schurink GW, Aarts NJ, Wilde J, et al: Endoleakage after stent-graft
    treatment of abdominal aneurysm: Implications on pressure imaging:
    An in vitro study. *J Vasc Surg* 28:234-241, 1998.

18. Mehta M, Ohki T, Veith FJ, et al: All sealed endoleaks are not the
    same: A treatment strategy based on an ex vivo analysis. *Eur J Vasc
    Endovasc Surg*, 21:541-544, 2001.

19. Gilling-Smith G, Brennan J, Harris P, et al: Endotension after endovas-
    cular aneurysm repair: Definition, classification, and strategies for
    surveillance and intervention. *J Endovasc Surg* 6:305-307, 1999.

CHAPTER 6

Endovascular Aortic Aneurysm Repair: Outcomes in Patients at Increased Risk for Standard Surgery

Peter H. Lin, MD
Assistant Professor of Surgery, Division of Vascular Surgery, Emory University School of Medicine, Atlanta, Ga

Ruth L. Bush, MD
Vascular Surgery Fellow, Division of Vascular Surgery, Emory University School of Medicine, Atlanta, Ga

Elliot L. Chaikof, MD, PhD
Associate Professor of Surgery, Division of Vascular Surgery, Emory University School of Medicine, Atlanta, Ga

With the advent of an endovascular treatment option for the abdominal aortic aneurysm (AAA), defining an appropriate strategy for the referral of patients to either open or endovascular repair remains a complex clinical endeavor. For example, patients who were otherwise appropriate surgical candidates for standard open repair have populated most, if not all, industry-sponsored clinical trials conducted in the United States.[1-3] Among these patients, a significant reduction in hospital stay has been demonstrated, with early return to preoperative levels of activity. Enthusiasm for endovascular treatment for the patient at low risk has also been coupled with the proposition that endovascular therapy provides an ideal approach for patients in whom standard operative repair carries an increased risk of perioperative morbidity and mortality.[4] Indeed, endovascular treatment has increased the proportion of patients now referred for AAA repair by providing therapy for patients who have been deemed inoperable because of the presence of significant comorbid conditions. Nonetheless, the widespread advocacy of endovascular grafting as a preferred option to open surgery for potentially all anatomically suitable patients continues during a period when most studies have reported outcomes that are largely confined to early intervals after intervention.

We recently reported the clinical experience with endovascular AAA repair at our institution.[5] This updated report reviews our midterm experience with endovascular AAA repair during a 7-year period by examining early and late clinical outcome in concurrent cohorts of patients stratified either as patients at low risk, who would otherwise be considered ideal open surgical candidates, or as those who are at increased risk for intervention. In these two groups of patients, we assessed perioperative morbidity and mortality, technical success, and late clinical success rates and patient survival.

MATERIALS AND METHODS

PATIENT SELECTION

Data for 236 consecutive patients undergoing elective endovascular AAA repair at Emory University Hospital (Atlanta, Ga) were retrospectively collected from April 1994 through March 2001. An endovascular program was initially instituted at Emory University as part of an investigator-sponsored, investigational trial (Endovascular Technologies, Inc, Menlo Park, Calif/Guidant, Inc, Indianapolis, Ind). This program expanded in 1999 to include a second investigational device (Excluder, WL Gore and Associates, Inc, Flagstaff, Ariz). We have also used the AneuRx (Medtronic, Inc, Sunnyvale, Calif) endograft system after its approval by the Food and Drug Administration for commercial use in September 1999. During the study period, implanted endografts included the EVT/Guidant endograft (n = 150), the AneuRx stent graft system (n = 58), and the Excluder endograft (n = 28). The EVT/Guidant endografts included tube (n = 26), bifurcated (n = 109), and aortoiliac endografts combined with a femorofemoral bypass graft (n = 15). The Gore endografts were all phase 2 devices.

Patients were considered at increased risk for intervention if there was (1) documentation of previous myocardial infarction (MI) or congestive heart failure, (2) significant respiratory disease as demonstrated by a forced expiratory volume in 1 second of less than 1 L/min or a requirement for home oxygen therapy, (3) chronic liver disease with documented cirrhosis or portal hypertension, or (4) the presence of concurrent or recent malignancy. Of note, all patients

underwent preoperative cardiac risk assessment that included dobutamine echocardiography or persantine thallium scanning.

ENDOGRAFT IMPLANTATION

All endovascular AAA repairs were performed in a standard operating department with complete angiographic capability by a team
of vascular surgeons and interventional radiologists. The techniques of transfemoral endovascular AAA prosthesis implantation
have been described previously.[1-4,6] Fluoroscopic guidance (OEC
9600, OEC Medical Systems, Inc, Thousand Oaks, Calif) was used
for placement of the endoprosthesis, and most of the procedures
were performed with the patients under general anesthesia. All
patients underwent systemic anticoagulation with heparin, 100
U/kg. Postimplantation aortography was performed to assess graft
positioning, vessel patency, periprosthetic leakage, and graft limb
stenosis. Type 1 endoleaks, leakage around the proximal or distal
attachment site, were treated during the operation with additional
endovascular measures. Type 2 endoleaks, those through retrograde lumbar or inferior mesenteric arteries, were observed and
monitored with serial computed tomography (CT) scans. At the
discretion of the attending physician, this type of endoleak was
treated with coil embolization of the patent collateral pathway.

CLINICAL FOLLOW-UP

Contrast-enhanced CT was performed either in the immediate postoperative period or within 1 month of endograft placement. Additional imaging studies including CT, duplex ultrasound scanning,
and plain abdominal x-ray evaluation were performed at 6 months,
12 months, and then annually thereafter. If an endoleak was visual-
ized, more frequent surveillance imaging was performed as clinically indicated.

DEFINITIONS

All perioperative complications are described; however, major morbidity was defined as any complication that resulted in an increase
in hospital stay, a secondary surgery, or a significant disability. The
definitions of technical success, clinical success, and continuing
success as described by the Society for Vascular Surgery/Interna-
tional Society for Cardiovascular Surgery (SVS/ISCVS) Ad Hoc
Committee on Reporting Standards for Endovascular AAA Repair
were used.[7] In brief, 30-day technical success was defined on an
intent-to-treat basis as successful endograft deployment without
death, need for standard aortic reconstruction for 30 days, or evi-

dence of persistent (>48 hours) endoleak. Clinical success was inclusive of those patients who at 6 months after implantation had spontaneously sealed a persistent endoleak and had demonstrated no evidence of aneurysm enlargement. Secondary clinical success was used if additional endovascular techniques were required to seal an endoleak. Continuing success was defined as the maintenance of both clinical and technical success without evidence of graft thrombosis, infection, endoleak, or aneurysm expansion of greater than 0.5 cm. Any late graft complication that was successfully treated by an endovascular technique was classified as a secondary continuing success. Other outcomes analyzed included successful graft deployment irrespective of the presence or absence of endoleak, surgical time, operative blood loss, duration of stay in an intensive care unit, length of hospital stay, and patient survival.

STATISTICAL ANALYSIS

Descriptive data are expressed as mean ± SD. Continuous variables were compared with the use of the Student t test. Nominal variables were analyzed by contingency tables. The Kaplan-Meier method with Mantel-Cox (log-rank) post hoc analysis was used to determine success and survival rates. $P < .05$ was considered statistically significant. An SAS statistical package was used for analysis (Version 5.0, Abacus Concepts, Berkeley, Calif).

RESULTS

Between April 1994 and March 2001, elective endovascular repair of infrarenal AAA was carried out on 236 patients, with 123 (52%) procedures conducted in patients classified as increased risk and 113 (48%) procedures performed in patients considered low risk for major morbidity or mortality. The incidence of comorbid conditions among patients deemed at increased risk for intervention is presented in Table 1. Patient and procedural characteristics for these two groups are summarized in Table 2, and the types of endografts implanted are described in Table 3.

Notably, cardiac disease was a major indication for the categorization of patients at increased risk for intervention. To obtain a more precise determination of the severity of cardiac disease in our population, additional risk stratification of patients was performed with the SVS/ISCVS Cardiac Grading System.[8] In brief, cardiac status is graded with a 0 to 3 flat scale where grade 0 indicates a patient with no symptoms and a normal electrocardiogram (ECG); grade 1 is used for a patient with no symptoms and a history of a remote MI (>6 months), occult MI by ECG, or fixed defect

TABLE 1.

Characteristics Defining Patients at Increased Risk for Intervention (n = 123)*

Characteristic	No (%)
Congestive heart failure	43 (35)
Myocardial infarction	74 (60)
Respiratory disease†	26 (21)
Chronic liver disease–cirrhosis/portal hypertension‡	7 (6)
Malignancy§	9 (7)

*Patients may have had more than one factor increasing the risk of intervention.
†Chronic obstructive pulmonary disease documented by pulmonary function testing with a forced expiratory volume in 1 second of less than 1 L/min or the need for home oxygen therapy.
‡Child's class B.
§Primary lung cancer (n = 5), metastatic colon cancer (n = 2; Duke's stage D), laryngeal cancer (n = 1), transitional cell carcinoma of the bladder (n = 1).

TABLE 2.

Comparison of Patient Subgroups Undergoing Endovascular AAA Repair

Characteristic	Increased-Risk Group (n = 123)	Low-Risk Group (n = 113)	P value
Age (y)	73.9 ± 9.2	72.1 ± 6.3	NS
AAA size (mm)	59.2 ± 13.3	51.2 ± 13.9	.007
Preprocedure serum creatinine level (mg/dL)	1.2 ± 0.5	1.1 ± 0.6	NS
Operative time (min)*	235 ± 95	219 ± 84	NS
Blood loss (mL)*	457 ± 432	351 ± 273	NS
Postoperative stay (d)*	4.8 ± 3.4	4.0 ± 3.9	NS
ICU stay (d)*	1.3 ± 1.8	0.5 ± 1.6	NS

Values are mean ± SD.
*Includes only patients having successful endograft deployment.
Abbreviations: AAA, Abdominal aortic aneurysm; *NS,* No statistical significance; *ICU,* intensive care unit.

TABLE 3.
Types of Endografts Implanted

Graft Type	Increased-Risk Group (n = 123)(%)	Low-Risk Group (n = 113)(%)
Bifurcated (Guidant)	54 (44)	52 (46)
Tube (Guidant)	9 (7)	19 (17)
Aortoiliac* (Guidant)	13 (11)	3 (2)
AneuRx (Medtronic)	37 (30)	21 (19)
Excluder (Gore)	17 (14)	11 (10)
Conversions†	3 (2)	6 (5)
Aborted procedures†	4 (3)	0 (0)

*Aortoiliac endograft performed in conjunction with contralateral common iliac artery occlusion and femorofemoral crossover graft.
†No significant difference when analyzed by Fischer exact test.

on dipyridamole thallium or similar scan; grade 2 is used for the patient with stable angina, the presence of a significant reversible perfusion defect on dipyridamole thallium scan, ejection fraction of 25% to 45%, controlled ectopy/arrhythmia, or compensated congestive heart failure; and grade 3 is used for patients with unstable angina, ejection fraction of less than 25%, symptomatic or poorly controlled ectopy/arrhythmia, poorly compensated or recurrent congestive heart failure, or MI within 6 months. Patients in the study classified as low-risk (n = 113) had an SVS/ISCVS cardiac score of 0, whereas patients categorized at increased risk solely by a history of cardiac disease had a score of 1.82 ± 0.53 (n = 71). Of note, most patients with cardiac disease had a score of 2 (58%; 41 of 71) or 3 (8%; 6 of 71).

TECHNICAL AND CLINICAL SUCCESS
Endovascular stent graft deployment was successful in 116 (94%) of 123 of patients at increased risk and in 107 (95%) of 113 patients at low risk, with conversion rates of 2.4% and 5.3%, respectively. No intraoperative deaths occurred. Intraoperative conversions to open repair or aborted procedures all occurred during attempted implantation of EVT/Guidant endografts except one case of attempted AneuRx endograft placement. These technical failures were not clustered during any given time period. In the increased-risk group, there were three immediate conversions to open repair and four aborted procedures. The sole case of AneuRx endograft conversion

occurred when a contralateral catheter was caught in the nitinol strut and was unable to be removed. In the second case of immediate conversion, the distal attachment hooks of an EVT/Guidant tube graft became caught on the aortic bifurcation and were unable to be released. In the third case, a device twist was not resolvable with endoluminal techniques. Two aborted procedure occurred in patients with tortuous, heavily calcified iliac arteries. One patient subsequently died of progressive congestive heart failure several weeks after hospital discharge, whereas the other patient declined open repair. The third and fourth aborted procedures were also related to an inability to access the aneurysm. The third patient declined open repair and subsequently had a fatal aneurysm rupture, and the fourth patient died 6 months later. The cause of death in this patient was not determined. A late conversion also occurred in this group at 30 months. A patient who underwent implantation with the original EndoVascular Grafting System (EVT, Inc) had attachment system failure in the form of a hook fracture. This was recognized because of the presence of a persistent endoleak and aneurysm enlargement.

The results for the low-risk group were similar, with six conversions. Two were related to iliac artery injury and two to inability to access the aneurysm because of narrowed and calcified iliac arteries. Two cases of EVT/Guidant device malfunction occurred during deployment. In all six cases that required conversion, successful open repair was performed without postoperative complications. Two late conversions occurred in the low-risk group, one a consequence of a hook fracture identified at 26 months and the other of a graft infection at 2 months.

The 30-day technical success rates as defined by the SVS/ISCVS reporting standards were 73% for the increased-risk group and 78% for the low-risk group (P = NS). At 1 month after implantation, 25 (20.3%) patients at increased risk and 21 (19.6%) at low risk had endoleaks detected by CT imaging. These results remained essentially unchanged at 6 months, with clinical success rates at 6 months of 83% for the patients at increased risk and 80% for the low-risk cohort. Thirteen patients at increased risk and five at low risk had spontaneous sealing of their endoleaks. All remaining endoleaks were observed during this period, and no further intervention was taken in this regard. Continuing primary and secondary success as defined by the SVS/ISCVS reporting standards are represented in Figure 1 and were approximately 77% at 24 months. Results were similar for both patient subgroups.

Adjunctive endovascular techniques were used in both groups to facilitate graft implantation and aneurysm exclusion. In 11 patients

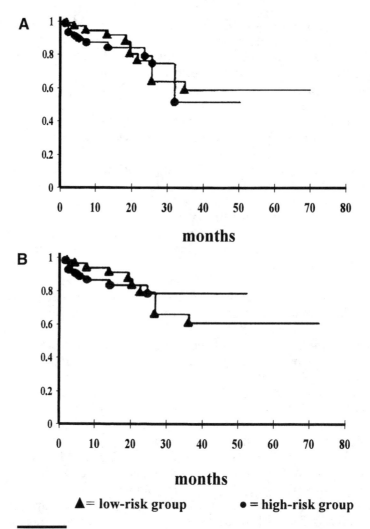

▲= low-risk group   ● = high-risk group

FIGURE 1.
Primary **(A)** and secondary **(B)** continuing success rates for low-risk *(solid triangles)* and increased-risk *(solid circles)* groups presented by Kaplan-Meier method. Statistically significant differences in success rates were not observed.

at increased risk, one or both limbs of a bifurcated graft had intraluminal stents placed for fabric folds observed with either intravascular ultrasound scanning or angiography at the time of endograft deployment. Intraluminal stents were also placed in 19 patients at low risk. Internal iliac arteries were unilaterally embolized in 13 patients (7 at high risk, 6 at low risk) for the exclusion of ectatic or aneurysmal common iliac arteries. Iliac artery dissection was noted in 1 patient in each study group at the time of graft implantation and was treated successfully in both cases with stent coverage.

COMPLICATIONS

The perioperative complication rate was 17.5% and 15.0% in the increased- and low-risk groups, respectively (Table 4). All wound infections were superficial and successfully treated on an outpatient basis with local wound care and antibiotic therapy. Two patients developed acute renal failure that required hemodialysis. Overall, major morbidity necessitating an increase in hospital stay or significant disability occurred in 4% (5 of 123) of patients at increased risk and 6% (7 of 113) of patients at low risk.

FOLLOW-UP

Follow-up data were complete for all patients, with a mean follow-up interval of 10.3 ± 13.8 months for patients at high risk and 21.3 ± 16.7 months for the low-risk group. No patient was lost to follow-up. The perioperative (30-day) mortality rates were 6.5% and 1.8% for the increased-risk and low-risk groups, respectively ($P =$ .2013, Fisher exact test). Eight perioperative deaths occurred in the group at increased-risk for intervention. One death occurred in a patient who required conversion from endovascular repair to open

TABLE 4.
Perioperative (30-Day) Complications

Complication	Increased-Risk Group (n = 120)	Low-Risk Group (n = 107)
Wound infection	11	8
Reexploration for hemostasis	2	3
Myocardial infarction	2	1
Renal failure (dialysis requirement)	1	1
Deep venous thrombosis/pulmonary embolism	0	2
Graft twist*	1	0
Common femoral artery injury	3	1
Pneumonia	1	0

*Twisting of one limb of a nonsupported bifurcated graft required treatment with a femorofemoral crossover graft at the time of stent graft implantation.

repair, and one in a patient who had an aborted procedure and severe coronary artery disease. The third death occurred in a patient who had a successful endovascular repair without evidence of postoperative endoleak. A malignant arrhythmia was the presumed cause of death. Two deaths occurred as a result of postoperative myocardial ischemia. One patient with severe chronic obstructive pulmonary disease and emphysema developed pneumonia postoperatively. He developed adult respiratory distress syndrome that eventually contributed to his death. The seventh patient developed acute renal failure and pneumonia postoperatively and died 2 weeks after the endovascular aneurysm repair. The eighth patient died of severe heart failure after hospital discharge. Endograft deployment had been successful in this patient, and no endoleak had been detected by CT scanning at the time of discharge. Fifteen other patients died during the follow-up period.

In the low-risk group, two perioperative and nine late deaths occurred. One death was caused by intraoperative hemorrhage, and another death occurred due to presumed postoperative pulmonary embolism. Kaplan-Meier cumulative survival curves are shown in Figure 2. The 2-year mortality rates were 26.5% ± 8.1% and 14.2% ± 7.5% for the increased- and low-risk groups, respectively. A significant difference between the two patient cohorts was noted by the Mantel-Cox (log-rank) test ($P = .035$). None of the reported late deaths in our series were related to the initial endovascular procedure, device failure, or late aneurysm rupture.

DISCUSSION

The introduction of endovascular grafting was a milestone in the treatment of patients with AAA in that it provided a treatment option for those patients with large aneurysms who had been deemed inoperable because of the presence of significant medical comorbidities.[4] In the extension of this technology to all patients with aneurysmal disease, clinical investigations have confirmed that compared with open surgery, an early benefit in quality of life can be achieved as it relates to reducing hospital stay and recovery period.[1,2] Nonetheless, even minimally invasive interventions may be associated with an adverse early outcome, and the presumption that an endovascular approach reduces perioperative mortality in patients at low risk compared with the results of standard surgery remains unproven. Moreover, an early benefit in quality of life may be offset by a lower level of late clinical success that carries with it a requirement for more intensive long-term surveillance, increased

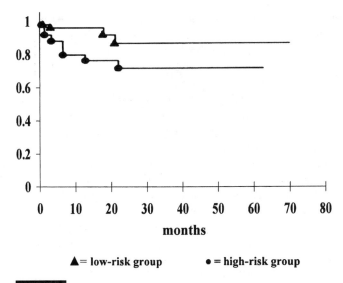

= low-risk group ● = high-risk group

FIGURE 2.
Cumulative survival rates for low-risk *(solid triangles)* and increased-risk *(solid circles)* groups presented by Kaplan-Meier method. A statistically significant difference in survival in favor of the low-risk group was noted by the log-rank test ($P < .035$).

rates of reintervention, and higher costs and psychological stress. Thus, in advocating endovascular treatment for patients who are at low risk for operative repair, a critical analysis of late outcomes is required.

In our retrospective analysis, patients classified at low risk for intervention with accepted clinical and laboratory criteria had a 30-day mortality rate of 1.8% after endovascular intervention. This result is of particular interest in the context of a recent review of open aortic surgery performed on 856 patients at our institution between 1986 and 1996.[9] The in- hospital mortality rate was 1.3%, with a major complication rate of 15.9%. Thus, although the data generated by these two distinct reviews at the Emory University Hospital are not strictly comparable, our experience suggests that in the patient at low risk, endovascular treatment of the infrarenal AAA is not associated with a reduction in perioperative mortality compared with standard surgical repair.

Many reports, nevertheless, confirm that endovascular strategies do offer unique advantages among those patients whose comorbid conditions increase the risk of major complications including death. For example, May et al[10] compared outcomes of patients treated concurrently with either open or endovascular repair. Although more than 40% of patients treated with endografts had been declined open repair because of comorbid illness, no significant difference in perioperative mortality rates or long-term survival was observed. In addition, Chuter at al[11] observed a 30-day mortality rate of 1.7% in their review of patients treated by endovascular approaches who had otherwise been refused conventional AAA repair. In their patient population, coronary artery disease was present in 81%, congestive heart failure in 34%, and respiratory disease in 49%. These reports compare favorably with published studies of conventional open aneurysmectomy in the patient at high risk that have been associated with mortality rates of up to 40%.[12-14]

Our review does reemphasize, however, that conversion to an open repair and the aborting of an endograft procedure may not be well tolerated among those patients with significant comorbidities. This is consistent with results reported by May et al,[10,15] who have noted mortality rates of 18% to 43% when primary conversion was required for patients considered at prohibitive risk for standard surgery. It is our view that the prolonged anesthesia time and the blood loss incurred during a preliminary attempt at endovascular repair before conversion are important contributing factors to these poor results. Therefore, a cautious approach should be adopted in recommending endovascular repair for the patient at high risk in the presence of anatomic constraints, which might reduce the potential for successful endograft deployment.

With SVS/ISCVS recommended reporting standards, 30-day primary technical success, 6-month clinical success, and 24-month primary and secondary continuing clinical success rates were all approximately 75% in both study subgroups. Our 30-day primary technical success rate is similar to the 77% rate reported by Zarins et al[2] for 190 patients treated as part of the multicenter Medtronic AneuRx stent graft trial. Likewise, our 24-month success rate is comparable to that recently reported by May et al[16] for second-generation endovascular prostheses used in 148 patients. Thus, although these results are encouraging and will undoubtedly improve in coming years, the success of endovascular repair remains uncertain in a significant proportion of patients. Two years after endograft implantation, 25% of all patients were classified as failures with the SVS/ISCVS reporting standards definition.[7] Therefore, in advocating an aggressive approach for endovascular intervention in the patient who is an otherwise ideal surgical candidate, it is also important to recognize that significant limitations to endovascular repair remain. Moreover, the impact of this failure rate on increasing costs and reducing patient quality of life is probably significant but admittedly was not defined in this report.

It is notable that all reported late deaths in our series were unrelated to the initial endovascular procedure, device failure, or late aneurysm rupture. Although late survival was significantly compromised in those patients who were deemed at increased risk for intervention, 75% were alive at 2 years. These results are not unexpected, and others have reported similar late mortality rates for patients initially considered poor surgical candidates.[11] Nonetheless, all of this suggests that the benefit of endovascular repair may be limited for patients who have a compromised life expectancy. In this regard, patients with a concomitant history of recent or concurrent malignant disease are a subgroup of particular interest. Of the nine patients in this group, two died of progressive cancer 12 months after endovascular AAA repair. However, the six remaining patients were alive at the time of last follow-up (12.4 ± 8.2 months). Thus, given the imprecision in predicting the risk of AAA rupture and long-term survival either in response to cancer therapy or other major medical illness, decisions to proceed with endovascular repair must be carefully individualized. In this regard, we presently advocate endovascular intervention for the patient with significant medical comorbidity only when aneurysm size is equal to or exceeds 6 cm in diameter and patient life expectancy is estimated to exceed 2 years. We believe this to be a prudent recommendation given respective annual rates of rupture of approximately 6.6% and 19% for untreated patients with 5.7-cm and 7.0-cm diameter aortic aneurysms[17] and our combined major morbidity and 30-day mortality rate of 12% for the patient at increased risk for intervention.

In summary, our analysis suggests that endovascular aneurysm repair currently remains most appropriate for those patients with large aneurysms who are otherwise prohibitive operative candidates. It is significant that endovascular grafting provides these patients with a treatment option when one was not previously available. Advocating endovascular treatment for the patient who is at low risk for standard operative intervention remains problematic. Although clinical success can be achieved in most patients, inadequate results continue to be observed in a significant proportion. In deciding on a course of treatment, an informed decision on the part of the patient requires a consideration of these data and an appreciation that endovascular aortic aneurysm repair remains in a relatively early stage of development.

REFERENCES

1. Moore WS, Rutherford RB: Transfemoral endovascular repair of abdominal aortic aneurysm: Results of the North American EVT phase 1 trial. EVT Investigators. *J Vasc Surg* 3:543- 553, 1996.
2. Zarins CK, White RA, Schwarten D, et al: AneuRx stent graft versus open surgical repair of abdominal aortic aneurysms: Multicenter prospective clinical trial. *J Vasc Surg* 29:292-308, 1999.
3. White RA, Donayre CE, Walot I, et al: Modular bifurcation endoprosthesis for treatment of abdominal aortic aneurysms. *Ann Surg* 226:381-391, 1997.
4. Parodi JC, Palmaz JC, Barone HD: Transfemoral intraluminal graft implantation for abdominal aortic aneurysms. *Ann Vasc Surg* 5:491-499, 1991.
5. Bush RL, Lumsden AB, Dodson TF, et al: Mid-term results after endovascular repair of the abdominal aortic aneurysm. *J Vasc Surg* 33:S70-S76, 2001.
6. Harris EJ: Modular systems in the treatment of abdominal aortic aneurysms: Lessons learned in the development of designer endografts. *Semin Vasc Surg* 12:170-175, 1999.
7. Ahn SS, Rutherford RB, Johnston KW, et al: Reporting standards for infrarenal endovascular abdominal aortic aneurysm repair. Ad Hoc Committee for Standardized Reporting Practices in Vascular Surgery of The Society for Vascular Surgery/International Society for Cardiovascular Surgery. *J Vasc Surg* 25:405-410, 1997.
8. Rutherford RB, Baker JD, Ernst C, et al: Recommended standards for reports dealing with lower extremity ischemia: Revised version. *J Vasc Surg* 26:517-538, 1997.
9. Berry A, Smith RB III, Weintraub W, et al: Age versus comorbidities as risk factors for complications after elective abdominal aortic reconstructive surgery. *J Vasc Surg* 33:345-352, 2001.
10. May J, White GH, Yu W, et al: Concurrent comparison of endoluminal versus open repair in the treatment of abdominal aortic aneurysms: Analysis of 303 patients by life table methods. *J Vasc Surg* 27:213-221, 1998.
11. Chuter TA, Reilly LM, Faruqi RM, et al: Endovascular aneurysm repair in high-risk patients. *J Vasc Surg* 31:122-133, 2000.
12. Sterpetti AV, Schultz RD, Feldhaus RJ, et al: Abdominal aortic aneurysm in elderly patients. Selective management based on clinical status and aneurysmal expansion rate. *Am J Surg* 150:772-776, 1985.
13. Morishita Y, Toyohira H, Yuda T, et al: Surgical treatment of abdominal aortic aneurysm in the high-risk patient. *Jpn J Surg* 21:595-599, 1991.
14. Hollier LH, Reigel MM, Kazmier FJ, et al: Conventional repair of abdominal aortic aneurysm in the high-risk patient: A plea for abandonment of nonresective treatment. *J Vasc Surg* 3:712-717, 1986.
15. May J, White GH, Yu W, et al: Conversion from endoluminal to open

repair of abdominal aortic aneurysms: A hazardous procedure. *J Vasc Surg* 14:4-11, 1997.

16. May J, White GH, Waugh R, et al: Comparison of first- and second-generation prostheses for endoluminal repair of abdominal aortic aneurysms: A 6-year study with life table analysis. *J Vasc Surg* 32:124-129, 2000.

17. Taylor LM, Porter JM: Basic data related to clinical decision-making in abdominal aortic aneurysms. *Ann Vasc Surg* 1:502-504, 1987.

PART III

Visceral Artery Disease

CHAPTER 7

Angioplasty and Stent Versus Surgical Reconstruction for the Treatment of Renal Artery Ostial Stenosis

Jennifer A. Heller, MD
Clinical Fellow, Division of Vascular Surgery, New York Presbyterian Hospital, Cornell Campus, New York, NY

K. Craig Kent, MD
Professor of Surgery, Weill Medical College of Cornell University, Chief, Division of Vascular Surgery, Director, Vascular Center, New York Presbyterian Hospital, New York, NY

Hypertension related to renal artery stenosis remains a prevalent and treatable condition that affects up to 2 million people in the United States. Moreover, renovascular occlusive disease is the suspected etiology of end-stage renal failure in up to 15% of the dialysis population.[1] The ability of renal revascularization, in appropriately chosen individuals, to alleviate hypertension and provide renal salvage has been carefully and repeatedly documented.

For more than 40 years, surgical reconstruction has been the mainstay of treatment for renovascular disease. Excellent outcomes have been repeatedly documented for surgical therapy regardless of the reconstructive technique. Surgical revascularization, however, has been largely replaced at many centers by catheter-based treatment of renal artery stenosis. The "less invasive" nature of catheter-based treatment of renal artery disease is appealing to both patients as well as their referring physicians. Moreover, a catheter-based approach to renal artery stenosis has allowed many physicians who traditionally refer their patients to surgeons to now be the primary interventionalist. In this chapter, we evaluate the available data regarding renal angioplasty and stent placement for ostial renal artery stenosis and compare the results of catheter-based treatments with those of surgical revascularization.

The first renal artery angioplasty was performed by Gruntzig et al[2] in 1978. A strong relationship between the location of disease in the renal artery and outcome of catheter-based interventions soon became apparent. Angioplasty is now established as a very effective treatment for most types of fibromuscular dysplasia, a disease process that is often focal and localized to the midsegment of the renal artery.[3] Even nonostial atherosclerotic lesions appear to respond well to renal artery angioplasty.[4] However, the preponderance of patients who have symptomatic renovascular disease are elderly with atherosclerosis as the cause. In these patients, disease is often found at or adjacent to the renal artery origin.

This distinction between ostial and nonostial renal artery lesions is clinically important. Ostial stenoses are derived from aortic (not renal) plaque that encroaches on and protrudes into the renal artery origin. Angioplasty produces its effect by fracturing and expanding (rather than compressing) atheromatous plaque. Thus, aortic plaque at the renal artery origin, which is oriented in a longitudinal rather than a circumferential fashion, is resistant to fracture and dilatation. There is often significant elastic recoil of ostial renal lesions after renal artery angioplasty. Moreover, the potential for dissection is increased when ostial stenoses are treated with angioplasty alone. As a consequence, both early and late outcomes for renal artery angioplasty of ostial renal artery lesions have been suboptimal.[5]

Arterial stents have evolved as a method of preventing elastic recoil and dissection. The use of stents for renal artery stenosis was first introduced by Palmaz et al[6] in 1987. The contribution of stents to the immediate technical outcome of angioplasty of disease at the renal artery origin subsequently became apparent. In 1999, van de Ven et al[7] reported the results of a randomized trial comparing the outcomes of angioplasty alone and angioplasty and stent for ostial renal artery stenosis. These investigators found an immediate patency of only 57% with angioplasty alone versus 88% with angioplasty and stent. At 6 months, patency rates associated with these two techniques remained markedly different (29% for angioplasty versus 75% for angioplasty and stent).

Although the techniques used for renal artery angioplasty and stent can vary, there are several salient features that deserve mention. Access is usually via the common femoral artery; however, a brachial approach can facilitate cannulation and manipulation of the renal vessels when there is substantial inferior angulation relative to the aorta. Balloon-expandable (vs self-expanding) stents are preferred because their greater radial force allows stabilization of aortic plaque. The renal artery may or may not be predilated depending on the severity of the renal artery stenosis. Precise placement of the stent relative to the aortorenal junction is crucial. The stent should be positioned at the renal artery ostium so that it extends at least 1 mm into the aortic lumen. This ensures that the aortic plaque, the primary cause of orificial narrowing, is effectively treated. The stent should be deployed with a balloon that expands to a diameter slightly greater than that of the normal distal renal artery. The initial technical end point (ie, the percent residual stenosis) is a critical predictor of the durability of this intervention; if a residual stenosis of more than 30% exists after the initial dilatation, redilatation should be considered (Fig 1).

During the past 10 years, more than 20 investigators have reported their results with either renal angioplasty or renal angioplasty and stent. Despite a large amount of data, clarity is lacking regarding the efficacy of these techniques. Several factors make analysis of these data difficult. In many of the reports, patients and techniques have not been properly segregated. Outcomes for patients who have hypertension and renal dysfunction as the indication for intervention are combined. Patients with ostial and nonostial lesions are

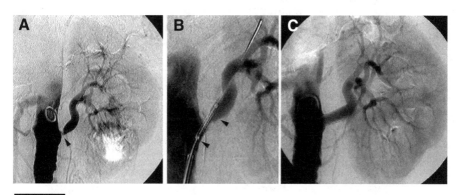

FIGURE 1.
A 58-year-old female with severe hypertension. **A,** Flush aortogram demonstrates severe ostial stenosis of the left renal artery *(arrowhead).* **B,** Stent in deployment position just before inflation *(arrowheads).* **C,** Conclusion of procedure, status-post stent deployment. (Courtesy of Trost DW, Sos TA, Pickering TG: Percutaneous transluminal angioplasty and stenting in renal artery stenosis: Renal artery thrombolysis. In Pollack HM, McClennan BL (eds). *Clinical Urography,* ed 2. Philadelphia, WB Saunders, 2000.)

often not distinguished despite the significant difference in the behavior of these lesions after treatment. In several studies, the outcome of patients treated with angioplasty and stent is combined with that of patients treated with angioplasty alone. Life tables are rarely used to report long-term results for patency, hypertension, or renal failure. Frequently, outcomes for hypertension and renal failure are not reported on a per patient basis, but rather an average blood pressure measurement or serum creatinine level is provided for the entire patient cohort. For example, the average creatinine level for a patient cohort may not change over time; however, within this cohort, there may be many individual patients who have either an increase or a decrease in their creatinine levels. This type of reporting can substantially limit our understanding of the data. There is extensive variability in the definition of an ostial lesion as well as the grading of stenoses. Lastly, follow-up of these patients is often poor or brief. The longest average follow-up for patients treated with renal artery angioplasty and stent is approximately 2.5 years as reported by Blum et al.[8] However, the average follow-up of all studies published during the past 10 years is only approximately 8 months.

With these reservations in mind, there is still a great deal of insight to be gained from recently reported trials. In Table 1, the results of several of the larger and more prominent series are displayed.[8-14] When evaluating these studies, it is important to consider the following variables: (1) immediate technical success, (2) 30-day procedural mortality and morbidity rates, (3) treatment of hypertension, (4) treatment of renal dysfunction, and (5) rate of restenosis.

The immediate technical success (defined in most trials as a residual stenosis < 30%) ranged from 88% to 100%. As is evident by these numbers, with experience and proper technique, excellent early outcomes are common. Major morbidity rates ranged from 6% to 50%; this wide range in frequency was related to the varying definitions of major complications. Significant complications related to renal artery angioplasty and stent include perinephric hematoma, arterial rupture, stent displacement, dissection, or acute arterial occlusion. Many of these technical complications, although major, are reversible. Dissections can be repaired with stents, and the patency of thrombosed renal arteries can be restored with thrombolysis (albeit renal damage may ensue after both events). The need for urgent surgical renal reconstruction after angioplasty and stent appears to be rare. Other complications include those related to the site of arterial access (eg, femoral pseudoaneurysm, hematoma, or arteriovenous fistula). Contrast-induced azotemia or

TABLE 1.
Results of Renal Artery Revascularization Outcome of Renal Artery Angioplasty and Stent

Study	Year	No. of Arteries	No. of Patients	Mean Age (y)	Initial Success (%)	Restenosis Rate (%)	Major Cx Rate (%)	Death Rate (%)	Mean F/U (mo)	Restenosis (%)	Hypertension (%)				Renal Failure (%)				
											Cured	Im-proved	No Change	Mean F/U (mo)	Cured	Im-proved	No Change	Worse	Mean F/U (mo)
Bakker[9]	1999	120	106	66	98	17	6	0	8.5		+	+	+	+	+	+	+	+	+
Rodriguez-Lopez[10]*	1999	125	108	72	98	5.5	7.2	3.2	+		13	55	32	+	0	0	96	4	+
van de Ven[11]	1999	52	42	66	88	14	17	0	6		15	43	43	6	0	12.5	65	23	6
Tuttle[12]	1998	148	129	71	98	14	4	2.7	8		2	53	45	+	0	13	76	11	+
Rundback[13]*	1998	54	45	70	94	26	4.4	4.4	12.5		+	+	+	+	0	19	47	33	3
Blum[8]	1997	74	68	60	100	15	0	0	27		16	62	22	27	0	0	100	0	27
White[14]*	1997	133	100	67	99	18.8	1	1	8.7		+	+	+	6	+	+	+	+	6

*Combined ostial and nonostial lesion population.

†Not delineated in the study.

Abbreviations: Cx, Complication; *F/U,* follow-up.

renal dysfunction related to cholesterol embolization (with or without the need for dialysis) also occurs with varying frequency (see below). Although potentially less frequent than with open surgical repair, renal angioplasty and stent may be complicated by myocardial infarction or stroke. The large number and variety of complications, however, serve to remind both interventionalists and patients that renal angioplasty and stent placement are not "noninvasive" procedures.

The 30-day mortality rate for these patients ranged from 0% to 4.4%. Interestingly, mortality rates for large surgical series (inclusive of patients who did not have concomitant aortic reconstruction) also range from 0% to 4.1%.[15-20] One must presume that in general, renal angioplasty and stent can be performed with mortality and morbidity rates less than those for open surgical repair. However, the relatively high mortality rates observed in several reports of catheter-based intervention demonstrate both the generally ill nature of patients who have renal artery stenosis as well as the stress associated with this intervention.

Outcomes regarding the long-term relief of hypertension after renal artery angioplasty and stent vary considerably. Cure of hypertension is unusual, as is the case in most series of surgical revascularizations. The percentage of patients who are cured or who have improvement of their hypertension after catheter-based interventions ranged from 43% to 78%. The follow-up period during which these results were accrued is short and varied from immediately after the procedure to 2.5 years. In general, renal angioplasty and stent placement appear to be less efficacious than surgery for the treatment of hypertension. Cure or improvement rates in surgical series ranged from 81% to 90%.[15-20] Moreover, in several reports of renal angioplasty and stent, relief of hypertension has not been durable. Tuttle et al[12] found immediately postprocedure a reduction from 2.2 to 1.8 in the number of blood pressure medicines required by a cohort of 129 patients treated with angioplasty and stent. However, at 6 months after these interventions, the average number of medicines per patient returned to the preoperative number.[8] Similar findings were reported by Iannone et al[21] and van de Ven et al.[22] Somewhat concerning is a recent report of 106 patients with hypertension and renal artery stenosis who were randomly assigned to undergo renal artery angioplasty or to receive antihypertensive drugs alone. Twelve months after angioplasty, there were no significant differences between the angioplasty and drug-therapy groups in systolic and diastolic blood pressures, daily drug doses, or renal function. Of note, only two of the angioplasty patients in this trial were treated with stents. Moreover, several of the medically treated patients crossed over to angioplasty during the course of the trial. Despite these reservations, the findings of this study underscore the need to prospectively validate the efficacy of renal artery angioplasty and stent in the treatment of hypertension, a task that has not yet been fully accomplished.[23]

There are two possible reasons for the diminished efficacy of renal artery angioplasty and stent in the alleviation of hypertension. The most obvious explanation is a high rate of restenosis after this intervention, leading to reversal of the beneficial effect provided by the initial dilatation. Embolization in some patient at the time of angioplasty may also produce peripheral ischemia and persistent hypertension. Alternatively, the diminished efficacy of catheter-based treatment for renal artery stenosis may be related to a lack of rigor by investigators in identifying patients whose hypertension is the direct result of renal artery disease. Both renal artery stenosis and hypertension are prevalent in elderly patients, and often the two are not related. A major and not completely solved task, is that of identifying in which patients renal artery stenosis is the cause of hypertension. In no reports of renal angioplasty and stent are there any descriptions of the methods used to prove a relationship between renal artery stenosis and hypertension. Institution of appropriate preoperative evaluation of these patients could potentially have a beneficial effect on the outcome of patients treated with catheter-based techniques.

A second potential beneficial outcome after renal angioplasty and stent is the stabilization or reduction of renal dysfunction. Alternatively, azotemia is a potential complication for patients with normal preintervention creatinine levels who are revascularized solely for the treatment of hypertension. In most reported series, the outcomes of patients with and without preexisting renal dysfunction are combined. Moreover, the outcomes of patients treated solely for ischemic nephropathy are seldom distinguished from those of patients treated for hypertension. Despite these general limitations, several studies provide useful data. Rundback et al[13] reported the outcome of 45 patients at two centers treated with angioplasty and stent for ischemic nephropathy. All of these patients had serum creatinine levels that were greater than 1.5 mg/dL. At 3 months, 19% of patients were improved, 47% were unchanged, and 33% worsened. These findings can be compared with the results of surgical revascularization for ischemic nephropathy. In 70 patients treated with renal artery reconstruction for ischemic nephropathy with a mean follow-up of 24 months, 49% of patients were improved, 36% patients were unchanged, and only 15% had worsening of renal function.[18]

Patients with renal artery stenosis who have hypertension as the indication for treatment may or may not have preexisting renal dysfunction. Dorros et al[24] found that in patients with normal preintervention creatinine levels, 5% had deterioration of renal function after angioplasty and stent, whereas in the group with preexisting renal failure, 45% had either transient or permanent azotemia. Van de Ven et al,[11] in a prospective, randomized study that included 42 patients with hypertension treated with angioplasty and stent, found that for patients with preexisting renal dysfunction, 28% had worsening of renal function after intervention, whereas for patients without preexisting renal failure, 8% developed azotemia. Alternatively, Hanson et al[18] reported that in patients with normal preprocedural creatinine levels treated with surgical revascularization, none developed azotemia postoperatively.

Microembolization or cholesterol embolization is a definite hazard associated with catheter manipulation of renal artery disease. The clinical history after microembolization, converse to that related to iodinated contrast, is of progressive and irreversible azotemia. Confirmation of the diagnosis is difficult in the absence of a renal biopsy; thus, the true incidence of this problem remains unknown. In patients with a functioning contralateral kidney, there could be significant renal damage related to embolization of the manipulated kidney without an overall change in a patient's serum creatinine level. A better understanding of this process and its frequency would be useful in defining the utility of catheter-based intervention for renovascular disease.

Identification of those patients who develop restenosis or thrombosis after renal artery angioplasty and stent has been inconsistent because of the lack of a reliable noninvasive method of evaluating renal artery anatomy. Blum et al[8] routinely performed angiography in a cohort of 68 patients treated with angioplasty and stent and identified a rate of restenosis, defined as greater than 50% luminal narrowing, of 11% with an average follow-up for these patients of 27 months. These relatively optimistic findings should be contrasted with rates of restenosis as high as 26% (6 months' follow-up) reported in other series in which postprocedural monitoring has been less rigorous.[13]

Although it is difficult to realistically compare data from independent trials of surgical and catheter-based renal revascularization, several generalizations can be made. Renal artery angioplasty and stent may have reduced procedural mortality and morbidity compared with open surgical repair, although the differences are not as significant as one might have anticipated. In any event, a catheter-based treatment of renal artery disease is intuitively more appealing to both patients and referring physicians. In a comparison of carotid endarterectomy versus carotid angioplasty and stent, it has been argued somewhat successfully that procedural costs, disability, and patient discomfort are not that dissimilar for the two procedures. In a comparison of surgical versus catheter-based renal revascularizations, this argument is more difficult to support. Even a "less invasive" extra-anatomic renal bypass requires either a flank or subcostal incision with a longer procedural time and hospital stay relative to a catheter-based procedure. Initial technical success is excellent for both surgical and catheter-based reconstructions. However, the durability and efficacy of surgical reconstruction appear to significantly supersede those of renal artery angioplasty and stent for both treatment of renal dysfunction and hypertension.

How should one clinically apply these data? The ideal surgical candidates will be those who can enjoy the long-term patency and clinical benefit of surgical revascularization. The 55-year-old otherwise healthy patient with few comorbidities should clearly be offered surgical reconstruction. Alternatively, the elderly, infirm patient with diffuse and severe atherosclerotic obliterans may achieve greater benefit from a shorter, albeit less durable, procedure. Patients with combined aortic and renal artery disease may benefit from simultaneous operative repair of both processes. However, because the addition of renal to aortic reconstruction has been shown to increase morbidity and mortality, it has been argued that patients with combined disease should have percutaneous treatment of their renal arteries before open aortic repair. For those patients who are neither young and healthy nor elderly and infirm, the most appropriate choice of interventions is less clear. Larger prospective studies of renal artery angioplasty and stent with longer follow-up will help to make these decisions.

Regardless of outcomes, it is likely at least for the immediate future, that market forces rather than the clinical science will be a significant driving force in the choice of treatments for renal artery stenosis. An increasing number of physicians have become involved in the catheter-based treatment of peripheral vascular disease, and the access of these physicians to patients will most certainly influence clinical practice. Renal angioplasty with stent placement is an exciting new approach to the treatment of renal artery disease. However, the responsibility is ours to prospectively validate this technique and gain a better understanding of its utility and durability in the treatment of this prevalent disease process.

REFERENCES

1. Hansen KJ: Renovascular disease, an overview, in Rutherford RB (ed): *Vascular Surgery*, ed 5. Philadelphia, WB Saunders, 2000, p 1593.
2. Gruntzig A, Kuhlmann K, Vereter W, et al: Treatment of renovascular hypertension with percutaneous transluminal dilatation of renal artery stenosis. *Lancet* 1:801-802, 1978.
3. Tegtmeyer CJ, Selby JB, Hartwell GD, et al: Results and complications of angioplasty in fibromuscular disease. *Circulation* 83:155S-161S, 1991.
4. Hoffman O, Carreres T, Sapoval M, et al: Ostial renal artery stenosis angioplasty: Immediate and mid-term angiographic and clinical results. *J Vasc Interv Radiol* 9:65-73, 1998.
5. Novick AC: Management of renovascular disease. A surgical perspective. *Circulation* 83:167S-171S, 1991.
6. Palmaz JC, Kopp DT, Hayashi H, et al: Normal and stenotic renal arteries: Experimental balloon-expandable intraluminal stenting. *Radiology* 164:705-708, 1987.
7. van de Ven PJG, Kaatee R, Beutler JJ, et al: Arterial stenting and balloon angioplasty in ostial atherosclerotic renovascular disease: A randomised trial. *Lancet* 353:282-286, 1999.
8. Blum U, Krumme B, Flugel P, et al: Treatment of ostial renal artery stenoses with vascular endoprostheses after unsuccessful balloon angioplasty. *N Engl J Med* 336:459-465, 1997.
9. Bakker J, Goffette PP, Henry M, et al: The Erasme Study: A multicenter study on the safety and technical results of the Palmaz stent used for the treatment of atherosclerotic ostial renal artery stenosis. *Cardiovasc Intervent Radiol* 22:468-474, 1999.
10. Rodriguez-Lopez JA, Werner A, Ray LI, et al: Renal artery stenosis treated with stent deployment: Indications, technique, and outcome for 108 patients. *J Vasc Surg* 29:617-624, 1999.
11. Van de Ven PJG, Kaatee R, Beutler JJ, et al: Arterial stenting and balloon angioplasty in ostial atherosclerotic renovascular disease: A randomised trial. *Lancet* 353:282-286, 1999.
12. Tuttle KR, Chouinard RF, Webber JT, et al: Treatment of atherosclerotic ostial renal artery stenosis with the intravascular stent. *Am J Kidney Dis* 32:611-622, 1998.
13. Rundback JH, Gray RJ, Rozenblit G, et al: Renal artery stent placement for the management of ischemic nephropathy. *J Vasc Interv Radiol* 9:413-420, 1998.
14. White CJ, Ramee SR, Collins TJ, et al: Renal artery stent placement: Utility in lesions difficult to treat with balloon angioplasty. *J Am Coll Cardiol* 30:1445-1450, 1997.
15. Cambria RP, Brewster DC, L'Italien GJ, et al: The durability of differ-

ent reconstructive techniques for atherosclerotic renal artery disease. *J Vasc Surg* 20:76-87, 1994.

16. Darling RC, Kreienberg PB, Chang BB, et al: Outcome of renal artery reconstruction: Analysis of 687 procedures. *Ann Surg* 230:524-532, 1999.
17. Hallett JW, Textor SC, Kos PB, et al: Advanced renovascular hyptertension and renal insufficiency: Trends in medical comorbidity and surgical approach from 1970 to 1993. *J Vasc Surg* 21:750-760, 1995.
18. Hansen KJ, Starr SM, Sands E, et al: Contemporary surgical management of renovascular disease. *J Vasc Surg* 16:319-331, 1992.
19. Reilly JM, Rubin BG, Thompson RW, et al: Long-term effectiveness of extraanatomic renal artery revascularization. *Surgery* 116:784-791, 1994.
20. Steinbach F, Novick AC, Campbell S, et al: Long-term survival after surgical revascularization for atherosclerotic renal artery disease. *J Urol* 158:38-41, 1997.
21. Iannone LA, Underwood PL, Nath A, et al: Effect of primary balloon expandable renal artery stents on long-term patency, renal function, and blood pressure in hypertensive and renal insufficient patients with renal artery stenosis. *Cathet Cardiovasc Diagn* 37:243-250, 1996.
22. Van de Ven PGJ, Beutler JJ, Kaatee R, et al: Transluminal vascular stent for ostial atherosclerotic renal artery stenosis. *Lancet* 346:672-674, 1995.
23. Van Jaarsveld BC, Krijnen P, Pieterman H, et al: The effect of balloon angioplasty on hypertension in atherosclerotic renal artery stenosis. *N Engl J Med* 342:1007-1014, 2000.
24. Dorros G, Jaff M, Jain A, et al: Follow-up of primary Palmaz-Schatz stent placement for atherosclerotic renal artery stenosis. *Am J Cardiol* 75:1051-1055, 1995.

PART IV

Access for Hemodialysis

CHAPTER 8

Vascular Access: The Utility of Cryopreserved Vein Allograft

Peter H. Lin, MD
Assistant Professor of Surgery, Division of Vascular Surgery, Emory University School of Medicine, Atlanta, Ga

Ruth L. Bush, MD
Vascular Surgery Fellow, Division of Vascular Surgery, Emory University School of Medicine, Atlanta, Ga

Victor J. Weiss, MD
Assistant Professor of Surgery, Division of Vascular Surgery, Emory University School of Medicine, Atlanta, Ga

Alan B. Lumsden, MD
Associate Professor of Surgery, Chief, Division of Vascular Surgery, Emory University School of Medicine, Atlanta, Ga

The prevalence of end-stage renal disease (ESRD) and the number of patients who require maintenance hemodialysis have risen steadily over the past two decades. According to the 1999 annual report of the United States Renal Data System (USRDS), more than 300,000 ESRD patients in the United States undergo maintenance hemodialysis annually.[1] Vascular access procedures account for more than 10% of the annual ESRD budget and are conservatively estimated at $1 billion annually.[1] Surgical procedures for hemodialysis access have become the most common vascular operation in this country today. The leading cause of morbidity in the ESRD patient population is related to vascular access placement and the resultant complications.[2,3]

Hemodialysis access placement patterns and ESRD patient characteristics have changed dramatically in the past two decades, according to the 1995 USRDS annual report.[2] As the average age of renal failure patients requiring dialysis has risen, patients who require hemodialysis access have more debilitated comorbid factors. Although the life expectancy on dialysis is increasing, the overall patency rates of hemodialysis access remain so dismal that it is anticipated each dialysis patient will require multiple dialysis access operations and revision procedures in their hemodialysis lifetime.

Since the radiocephalic autogenous arteriovenous (AV) fistula was first introduced in 1965 by Brescia et al,[4] it remained the preferred hemodialysis access choice, in part because of its simplicity, durability, and relatively low complication rates. In addition, matured autologous AV fistulas have superior patency rates compared with those of prosthetic AV grafts. However, in a treatment guideline published by the National Kidney Foundation entitled the *Dialysis Outcome Quality Initiative*,[5] an increased number of hemodialysis AV graft operations were being performed compared with primary AV fistulas, presumably due in part to the increased age of dialysis patients who lack the superficial venous anatomy necessary for primary AV fistulas. Other reports also noted that prosthetic polytetrafluoroethylene (PTFE) AV grafts were constructed almost twice as often as autologous AV fistulas.[6] Among the common complications related to prosthetic AV grafts, which include infection, pseudoaneurysm, and graft thrombosis, prosthetic AV graft infection remains one of the most formidable challenges in the care of hemodialysis patients. General therapeutic principles include infected AV graft removal, appropriate intravenous antibiotic therapy, wide debridement and drainage, followed by placement of either a hemodialysis catheter or AV graft placement elsewhere in the body. With these multiple revision procedures, available access sites in the upper extremities will become scarce. The use of alternative strategies to maintain continuous hemodialysis access in the upper extremities, particularly in an infected field, becomes critically important.

Recent interest has arisen in the use of cryopreserved vein allograft as a conduit in the management of difficult hemodialysis access.[7-10] Clinical studies of cryopreserved allograft have received close scrutiny in the field of lower extremity vascular reconstruction, particularly in the infected area.[11,12] The concept of fresh venous allograft used as a vascular conduit was first introduced by Carrell in 1912 in which aortic replacement was performed in canine studies.[13] The clinical application of fresh allograft in humans was reported by Linton in 1955.[14] Shortly after that, efforts were made to preserve vein to allow for prolonged duration of storage so that venous allografts could be readily available for vascular reconstruction.[15] In the last two decades, clinical experience with the use of cryopreserved vein allograft has continued to increase, presumably because of the refinement of cryopreservation techniques and the availability of these allografts through commercial ventures.

METHOD OF CRYOPRESERVATION

The primary goal of tissue cryopreservation is to provide vein graft availability with minimal antigenicity as well as viable functional and structural integrity. Several organ procurement agencies, such as CryoLife, Inc (Kennesaw, Ga) and Northwest Tissue Center (Seattle, Wash), which follow the tissue preservation requirement set forth by the American Association of Tissue Banks and the United Network for Organ Sharing, provide cryopreserved vein allografts for vascular reconstruction. Before cryopreservation, all allografts are tested for communicable fungal, bacterial, and viral disease (ie, hepatitis A, B, C, human immunodeficiency virus types 1 and 2). Because the effect of cryopreservation on viral inactivation remains unclear, there is a theoretical, albeit small risk of viral disease transmission with the use of cryopreserved allograft. With more than 40,000 cryopreserved allograft implants worldwide, however, there has been no known case of viral or bacterial transmission associated with the use of cryopreserved allograft.

Although multiple techniques have been used for vein graft preservation, a common method is to harvest saphenous vein or femoral vein from organ donors within 24 hours after cessation of circulation. Careful surgical techniques are followed to maintain the structural integrity of the vein graft. The vein graft is placed in cryoprotectants and stored in the vapor phase of liquid nitrogen between $-110°C$ and $-196°C$. Without cryoprotectants, an intracellular vapor gradient is created when the extracellular matrix freezes at $0°C$. Under such a condition, the cytoplasm remains in a liquid form that could lead to cellular membrane disruption, resulting in nonviable and structurally damaged vein conduits.[16-18] In a study by Stephen et al[19] in which saphenous vein allografts were harvested without cryoprotectants and implanted as arterial conduits, a graft failure rate of 90% occurred in 6 months. With the use of cryoprotectants, the intracellular vapor gradient is minimized, which prevents membrane disruption during the freezing process. Commonly used cryoprotectants include dimethyl sulfoxide (DMSO), either in 10% or 20% concentration, and chondroitin sulfate.[20,21]

FUNCTIONAL CHARACTERISTICS AND ANTIGENICITY OF THE CRYOPRESERVED VEIN

Although several morphologic studies have documented an intact endothelium layer in cryopreserved vein allografts,[20-22] numerous animal studies have shown moderate endothelial denudation of cryopreserved vein allografts after implantation in the arterial circulation.[21,22] Clinical studies in humans showed a similar loss of endothelial layer in the cryopreserved saphenous vein allograft after arterial implantation, presumably due in part to a more rapid accumulation of low-density lipoprotein cholesterol compared with noncryopreserved human saphenous vein grafts.[23] The antithrombotic properties, platelet deposition, and fibrinolytic activities remained intact in the cryopreserved vein grafts.[24-26] Elmore et al[26] examined the functional status of the cryopreserved saphenous vein allograft implanted in canine femoral arteries and found similar contractile characteristics and graft patency rates compared with noncryopreserved saphenous vein grafts. However, there was a decrease in smooth muscle cell relaxation in response to nitric oxide in the cryopreserved vein grafts. Miller et al[27] examined the functional properties of the cryopreserved smooth muscle cells in organ chambers and noted a decreased contractile response to phenylephrine and endothelin. The decreased contractile response of the cryopreserved smooth muscle cells may be caused in part by the eventual replacement of the smooth muscle cell layer by fibrotic layers after cryopreserved allograft implantation.[11,15,27-29]

Several studies found cryopreserved vein allografts remained antigenic, since cryopreservation did not significantly affect the allograft antigenicity.[30-32] In an effort to decrease the antigenicity, several investigators noted adjunctive immunosuppression was beneficial in decreasing antigenicity and improving cryopreserved allograft patency in animal studies.[27,33-35] Posner et al[36] used a combination of immunosuppressants (cyclosporine, azathioprine, prednisone) and anticoagulants (warfarin, aspirin) plus vasodilators and noted an improved patency in the cryopreserved saphenous vein graft in humans. In contrast, a recent study by Carpenter and Tomaszewski[37] noted no significant benefit of immunosuppression in cryopreserved saphenous vein allograft patency in humans.

Baraldi et al[38] evaluated the immunologic status in 16 patients who underwent cryopreserved saphenous vein allografts for hemodialysis access and compared them with 17 patients with PTFE hemodialysis AV grafts. They found no significant difference in T-cell subpopulations, including CD3, CD4, and CD8 counts, or lymphocytotoxic antibodies between the two patient groups. Moreover, immunohistochemical examination of the cryopreserved hemodialysis AV graft showed minimal mononuclear cell infiltration in the adventitial allograft layer. The authors concluded that implantation of cryopreserved saphenous vein graft as hemodialysis access does not elicit significant immunologic activation or clinical rejection.[38] In contrast, several recent studies have demonstrated allosensitization in patients who received cryopreserved vein allografts for hemodialysis AV access, as evidenced by increased panel reactive antibody levels.[39,40] This allosensitization precluded renal transplantation in these hemodialysis patients. It was postulated that the allosensitization in these nonimmunosuppressed patients was caused in part by the exposure to allogenic class I and II major histocompatibility complex (MHC) antigens present on the cryopreserved endothelial cells. To address the issue of potential allosensitization to the cryopreserved endothelial cells, a new cryopreserved femoral vein allograft (CryoVein SG, CryoLife, Inc) has been developed that enzymatically removes the native endothelial cells but maintains the collagen matrix, which allows the recipient's own endothelial cells to repopulate the collagen matrix.[41] A prospective multicenter study is currently underway to examine the effect of alloimunization and patency rate in patients with endothelium-depleted cryopreserved vein allograft for hemodialysis access.

SURGICAL TECHNIQUE

Cryopreserved saphenous vein or femoral vein allograft can be ordered through several commercial sources and shipped overnight to any hospital in the United States. Specific ABO blood-type compatibility is recommended to avoid antigenic response between the donor allograft and the recipient. The cryopreserved allograft can be stored in dry ice packing for up to 72 hours, which maintains cellular viability of the allograft. To prepare the cryopreserved vein allograft, it is first submerged in a warm water bath (37°C-42°C) that rapidly thaws the allograft without adversely affecting cellular viability. The allograft is further prepared using a series of solution provided by the manufacturer (CryoLife, Inc) before it is ready for implantation (Fig 1).

A cryopreserved femoral vein allograft is usually less than 25 cm in length with a diameter ranging from 5 to 7 mm. Because of the limitation of the allograft length, it is recommended that the distance between the arterial and venous anastomotic sites be determined first to ensure that it is less than the cryopreserved femoral vein length. We routinely administer 3000 units of heparin systemically before clamping the axially vein. It is important to irrigate the cryopreserved allograft with heparinized saline solution to ensure that the antegrade flow direction of the vein allograft is maintained. In the case of an infected prosthetic brachial-axillary AV graft, the cryopreserved vein allograft may be placed in the infected field after the removal of the infected AV graft. However, we advocate tunneling the cryopreserved vein allograft away from the infected field (Fig 2). We prefer to perform the venous anastomosis first using running 6-0 polypropylene sutures. The venous end of the cryopreserved allograft is beveled to create an oblique end-to-side anastomosis of 7 or 8 mm in size to the axillary vein (Fig 3). Once the venous anastomosis is completed, venous clamps may be released from the axillary vein. It is not necessary to place a vascular clamp on the allograft while arterial anastomosis is constructed because the valves within the allograft will prevent any backbleeding (Fig 3). The arterial anastomosis is similarly constructed using 6-0 polypropylene sutures. The arterial end of the allograft is intentionally tapered to create an anastomosis of 4 mm in the brachial artery in an end-to-side fashion (Fig 4). The overlying connective tissue and skin are closed using absorbable polyglactin sutures. The cryopreserved brachial-axillary AV graft is allowed 3 to 4 weeks to mature before it is accessed for hemodialysis (Fig 5).

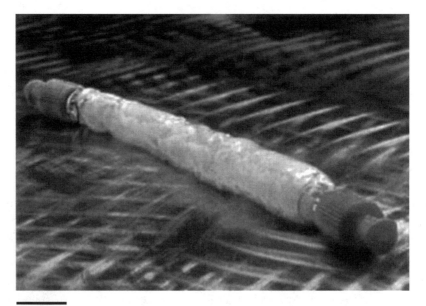

FIGURE 1.
The cryopreserved femoral vein allograft (CryoVein, CryoLife, Inc).

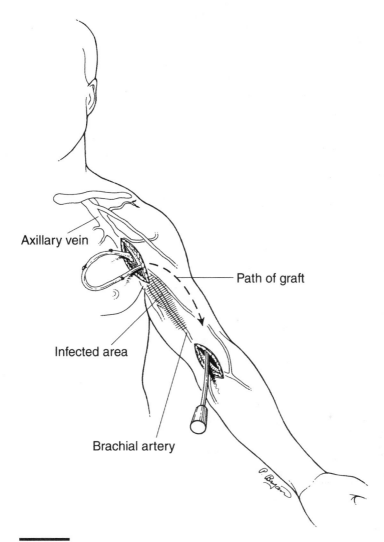

Axillary vein

Path of graft

Infected area

Brachial artery

FIGURE 2.
The cryopreserved vein allograft, which is tunneled away from the infected area, is used to construct a brachial-axillary hemodialysis AV graft.

CLINICAL EXPERIENCE

Baraldi et al[9] compared the function and patency rates in two groups of patients with AV fistulas constructed with either fresh saphenous veins (n = 35) or cryopreserved saphenous vein allografts (n = 32).[9] Functional analysis with punched biopsy of the AV fistula demonstrated a decreased production of 6-keto pros-

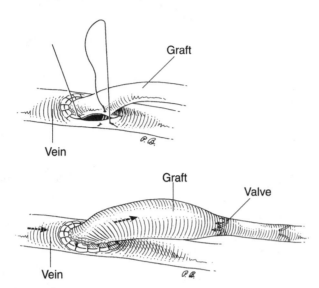

FIGURE 3.
The venous anastomosis is performed in an end-to-side fashion in the axillary vein. The venous valves within the cryopreserved allograft prevent any backbleeding, and vascular clamping is not necessary while the arterial anastomosis is constructed.

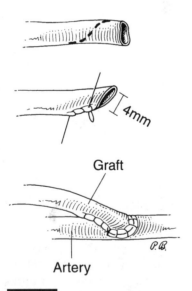

FIGURE 4.
The arterial end of the cryopreserved allograft is tapered to create a 4-mm anastomosis in the brachial artery.

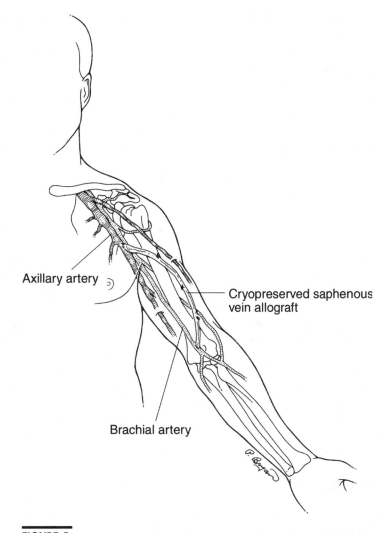

FIGURE 5.
The completed brachial-axillary cryopreserved AV graft is allowed 3 to 4 weeks to mature before it is accessed for hemodialysis.

taglandin F_{1a} and endothelial-derived relaxing factor in the cryopreserved AV allograft. In the fresh saphenous vein group, the prostaglandin production was stimulated by arachidonic acid and bradykinin. However, the prostaglandin production remained unresponsive to stimulation in the cryopreserved vein group. Clinical patency rates at 1 year remained similar between the two groups, with 82% in the fresh saphenous vein group and 72% in the cryopreserved vein group.[9]

Takamoto et al[42] examined the utility of cryopreserved femoral arterial allograft as hemodialysis access in five patients. Routine lymphocyte subset analysis and total lymphocyte count, and human leukocyte antigen class 1 antigen-antibody analysis were performed in the first 2 years after implantation, which demonstrated a weak activation in the immunologic lymphocyte markers. Moreover, histologic examination showed infiltration of inflammatory cells in the allograft wall, suggestive of minor immunologic reactions in the allograft. Nonetheless, the overall graft patency rates remained excellent, with 1- and 2-year graft patency rates of 100% and 84%, respectively.[42]

Matsuura et al[7] performed a prospective study of 44 patients undergoing 48 cryopreserved femoral vein AV grafts. Among them, 20 patients had prosthetic AV graft infections with no available contralateral venous access; 14 patients had ongoing bacteremia elsewhere in the body, which contraindicated a new prosthetic AV graft placement; and 10 patients had compromised venous outflow in whom cryopreserved femoral vein grafts were placed as the last surgical option. The 12-month primary patency and secondary rates were 49% and 75%, respectively, which were similar to those of the control group of PTFE AV grafts. The authors noted that cryopreserved femoral AV grafts could tolerate standard graft revision and thrombectomy in efforts to prolong the patency rate. In addition, the authors noted that despite the majority of their patients having bacteremia or an infectious source at the time of cryopreserved AV graft placement, no subsequent infection occurred in either initially infected operative sites or cryopreserved femoral vein AV grafts in their 3-year follow-up period. Based on their findings, the authors concluded that the cryopreserved femoral vein could be implanted safely and have an acceptable patency rate in the presence of infection, with a low risk of recurrent infection.

During the past 3 years at out institution, we have placed 26 cryopreserved femoral vein allografts in 24 patients with difficult hemodialysis access. The indications for cryopreserved femoral vein AV allograft included infected prosthetic AV graft replacement in 14 patients, remote bacteremia or sepsis in 8 patients, and compromised outflow central veins in 2 patients. The 1-year cumulative patency rate of cryopreserved femoral vein AV allografts was 68%, which was similar to the patency rate of prosthetic AV grafts previously reported from our institution.[43] Although no recurrent infections occurred in those with remote bacteremia or whose infected AV grafts were replaced with cryopreserved femoral vein allografts, 1 patient developed aneurysmal degeneration in the cryopreserved femoral vein AV allograft near the puncture access site 14 months after the allograft implantation. In our experience, cryopreserved femoral vein allograft is an effective alternative for patients with difficult hemodialysis access, such as those with prosthetic AV graft infection or ongoing bacteremia.

CONCLUSION

Cryopreserved vein allograft is an acceptable graft conduit in difficult hemodialysis access situations. Implantation of cryopreserved vein allograft elicits no significant clinical evidence of allograft rejection. The risk of recurrent infection remains exceedingly low when the cryopreserved allograft is used in the setting of prosthetic AV graft infection. Furthermore, the 2-year patency rates of cryopreserved vein AV grafts remain comparable to those of standard prosthetic AV grafts. With the excellent results in available clinical studies, the cryopreserved vein allograft is a durable hemodialysis access conduit and represents an exciting new alternative for treating patients with difficult hemodialysis access.

REFERENCES

1. The United States Renal Data System 1999 annual data report. *Am J Kidney Dis* 34:S1-S176, 1999.
2. The United States Renal Data System 1996 annual data report. *Am J Kidney Dis* 28:S1-S165, 1996.
3. Feldman HI, Held PJ, Hutchinson JT, et al: Hemodialysis vascular access morbidity in the United States. *Kidney Int* 43:1091-1096, 1993.
4. Brescia MJ, Cimino JE, Appel K, et al: Chronic hemodialysis using venipuncture and a surgically created arteriovenous fistula. *N Engl J Med* 275:1089-1092, 1966.
5. Schwab S, Besarab A, Beathard G: *Clinical Practice Guideline for Vascular Access. National Kidney Foundation, Dialysis Outcome Quality Initiative.* New York, National Kidney Foundation, 1997, pp 15-33.
6. Eknoyan G, Levin N: Implementation of NKF-DOQI: A progress report. *Nephrol News Issues* 13:11-15, 43, 1999.
7. Matsuura IH, Johansen KH, Rosenthal D, et al: Cryopreserved femoral vein grafts for difficult hemodialysis access. *Ann Vasc Surg* 14:50-55, 2000.
8. Matsuura IH: Cryopreserved human femoral vein: A new option for infected access grafts. *Contemp Dial Nephrol* Nov:30- 32, 1999.
9. Baraldi A, Bonucchi D, Di Felice A, et al: Liquid nitrogen snap frozen saphenous vein for vascular access in dialysis. *ASAIO Trans* 37:M225-M227, 1991.

10. Matsuura IH, Rosenthal D: The role of cryopreserved femoral vein graft in hemodialysis access surgery. *Perspect Vasc Surg* 13:71-80, 2000.

11. Fujitani RM, Bassiouny HS, Gewertz BL, et al: Cryopreserved saphenous vein allogenic homografts: An alternative conduit in lower extremity arterial reconstruction in infected fields. *J Vasc Surg* 15:519-526, 1992.

12. Shah RM, Faggioli GL, Mangione S, et al: Early results with cryopreserved saphenous vein allografts for infrainguinal bypass. *J Vasc Surg* 18:965-971, 1993.

13. Carrell A: Ultimate results of aortic transplantations. *J Exp Med* 15:389-392, 1912.

14. Linton R: Some practical considerations in the surgery of blood vessel grafts. *Surgery* 38:817-834, 1955.

15. Barner HB, DeWeese JA, Schenk EA: Fresh and frozen homologous venous grafts for arterial repair. *Angiology* 17:389- 401, 1966.

16. Litvan GG: Mechanism of cryoinjury in biological systems. *Cryobiology* 9:182-191, 1972.

17. Dent TL, Weber TR, Lindenauer SM, et al: Cryopreservation of vein grafts. *Surg Forum* 25:241-243, 1974.

18. Weber TR, Dent TL, Salles CA, et al: Cryopreservation of venous homografts. *Surg Forum* 26:291-293, 1975.

19. Stephen M, Sheil AG, Wong J: Allograft vein arterial bypass. *Arch Surg* 113:591-593, 1978.

20. Showalter D, Durham S, Sheppeck R, et al: Cryopreserved venous homografts as vascular conduits in canine carotid arteries. *Surgery* 106:652-659, 1989.

21. Brockbank KG, Donovan TJ, Ruby ST, et al: Functional analysis of cryopreserved veins. Preliminary report. *J Vasc Surg* 11:94-102, 1990.

22. Faggioli GL, Gargiulo M, Giardino R, et al: Long-term cryopreservation of autologous veins in rabbits. *Cardiovasc Surg* 2:259-265, 1994.

23. Ligush J, Berceli SA, Moosa HH: First results on the functional characterictics of cryopreserved human saphenous vein. *Cells and Materials* 1:359-368, 1991.

24. Malone JM, Moore WS, Kischer CW, et al: Venous cryopreservation: Endothelial fibrinolytic activity and histology. *J Surg Res* 29:209-222, 1980.

25. Bambang LS, Mazzucotelli JP, Moczar M, et al: Effects of cryopreservation on the proliferation and anticoagulant activity of human saphenous vein endothelial cells. *J Thorac Cardiovasc Surg* 110:998-1004, 1995.

26. Elmore JR, Gloviczki P, Brockbank KG, et al: Cryopreservation affects endothelial and smooth muscle function of canine autogenous saphenous vein grafts. *J Vasc Surg* 13:584-592, 1991.

27. Miller VM, Bergman RT, Gloviczki P, et al: Cryopreserved venous allografts: Effects of immunosuppression and antiplatelet therapy on patency and function. *J Vasc Surg* 18:216-226, 1993.

28. Balderman SC, Montes M, Schwartz K, et al: Preparation of venous allografts. A comparison of techniques. *Ann Surg* 200:117-130, 1984.
29. Bank HL, Schmehl MK, Warner R, et al: Transplantation of cryopreserved canine venous allografts. *J Surg Res* 50:57-64, 1991.
30. Axthelm SC, Porter JM, Strickland S, et al: Antigenicity of venous allografts. *Ann Surg* 189:290-293, 1979.
31. Nataf P, Guettier C, Hadjiisky P, et al: Evaluation of cryopreserved arteries as alternative small vessel prostheses. *Int J Artif Organs* 18:197-202, 1995.
32. Cochran RP, Kunzelman KS: Cryopreservation does not alter antigenic expression of aortic allografts. *J Surg Res* 46:597-599, 1989.
33. Schmitz-Rixen T, Megerman J, Colvin RB, et al: Immunosuppressive treatment of aortic allografts. *J Vasc Surg* 7:82-92, 1988.
34. Augelli NV, Lupinetti FM, el Khatib H, et al: Allograft vein patency in a canine model. Additive effects of cryopreservation and cyclosporine. *Transplantation* 52:466-470, 1991.
35. Pefioff LJ, Reckard CR, Rowlands DT, et al: The venous homograft: An immunological question. *Surgery* 72:961-970, 1972.
36. Posner MP, Makhoul RG, Altman M, et al: Early results of infrageniculate arterial reconstruction using cryopreserved homograft saphenous conduit (CADVEIN) and combination low-dose systemic immunosuppression. *J Am Coll Surg* 183:208-216, 1996.
37. Carpenter JP, Tomaszewski JE: Immunosuppression for human saphenous vein allograft bypass surgery: A prospective randomized trial. *J Vasc Surg* 26:32-42, 1997.
38. Baraldi A, Manenti A, Di Felice A, et al: Absence of rejection in cryopreserved saphenous vein allografts for hemodialysis. *ASAIO Trans* 35:196-199, 1989.
39. Benedetto B, Lipkowitz J, Madden R, et al: Use of cryopreserved cadaver vein allograft precludes renal transplantation due to allosensitization. Abstract presented at 33th Annual American Society of Nephrology Meeting, Toronto, October 2000.
40. Millers G, Lipkowitz J, Devivo J, et al: Alloimunization after cryopreserved allograft vein transplant. Abstract presented at American Society of Histocompatability Meeting, Orlando, Fla, October 2000.
41. CryoLife Inc, Clinical Research Department of Communication, 2001.
42. Takamoto S, Nakajima S, Okita Y, et al: Cryopreserved femoral arterial allografts for vascular access in hemodialysis. *Transplant Proc* 30:3917-3919, 1998.
43. Lumsden AB, MacDonald MJ, Isiklar H, et al: Central venous stenosis in the hemodialysis patient: Incidence and efficacy of endovascular treatment. *Cardiovasc Surg* 5:504-509, 1997.

PART V

Venous Disease

CHAPTER 9

Endovenous Saphenous Vein Ablation

John J. Bergan, MD, FACS, FRCS (Hon) Eng
Clinical Professor of Surgery, University of California, San Diego;
Clinical Professor of Surgery, Uniformed Services University of the
Health Sciences, Bethesda, Md

Primary venous insufficiency and varicose veins are an important vascular condition. In Western civilization, 15% of men and 25% to 50% of women are affected, and nearly all the women are symptomatic with aching leg pain, leg fatigue, night cramps, burning pain of venous neuropathy, and focal itching, which precedes dermatitis.[1] Varices have a multifactorial etiology that includes a hereditary substrate, female gender, pregnancy, and female hormones in general and progesterone in particular.[2,3] The fundamental pathophysiologic process is venous reflux, which commonly is confined to the superficial system of veins, but may be accompanied by deep venous system reflux[4] and perforating vein incompetence.[5] Thrombotic obstruction of veins may be important in individual cases, but reflux may still be the dominant cause of symptoms.

Treatment of primary venous insufficiency involves removing malfunctioning venous segments from the circulation.[6] In practice, this consists of two different maneuvers. The first removes the refluxing greater saphenous vein from the circulation, and the second excises elongated and stretched varicose veins.[7] These are two separate and distinct operative procedures even though they are usually performed in the same operative setting using the same anesthetic. The first carries CPT code 37720 and the second, 37785. Failure to correct saphenous reflux is a major cause of recurrent varicose veins after any type of intervention.[8,9]

SURGERY OF THE SAPHENOUS VEIN

Several options are available for removing the saphenous vein from the circulation (Table 1). Saphenous ligation at the saphe-

TABLE 1.

Options in Saphenous Vein Surgery

Saphenofemoral junction ligation
Saphenous vein stripping
  Ankle to groin
  Groin to knee
Sclerotherapy ablation
  Blind cutaneous puncture
  Ultrasound-guided sclerosant
  Sclerosant foam
Electromagnetic energy
  Radiofrequency energy
  Laser light energy

---

nofemoral junction with ligation of all tributary vessels but without saphenous removal (termed crossectomy in Europe) has been widely practiced but has consistently failed to prevent recurrent varices as compared with stripping out the saphenous vein in its thigh portion.[10] Of course, recurrence of varices may result from any of a number of causes alone or in combination. The one that we are concerned with in this discussion is failure to ablate the saphenous vein in its thigh portion. Relevant to that is the theory of neovascularization in which superficial recurrent groin varices are thought to communicate directly with the common femoral vein.[11]

Traditional teaching has held that evaluation of the results of varicose vein surgery required, at the very least, an observation period of 5 years. Two elements have changed that view. The first is the advent of duplex scanning. The duplex ultrasound scanner can evaluate saphenous patency, flow, and reflux as early as the immediate postprocedure interval and as late as the patient agrees to return. Repetitive examinations are patient acceptable. Thus, failures of total saphenous removal can be detected early.

The second element is developing knowledge that limbs that are re-forming recurrent or persistent varices have usually done so within the first year. For example, the 5-year report of Dwerryhouse et al,[12] which described a prospective, randomized comparison of groin-to-knee saphenous stripping with ligation and division of the saphenofemoral junction, revealed markers of early varix recurrence. A third of those limbs that would redevelop reflux, and 8 of 11 limbs with recurrent varicosities had demonstrated these by 1 year after the incident surgery.[13] In the report by

Sarin et al,[9] 43 limbs were assessed 21 months after saphenous stripping. The incidence of recurrent varicosities was 29% and that of recurrent reflux was 49%. In these limbs, 9 of the 21 had shown this reflux as early as 3 months after stripping.

Duplex scanning has the capability of separating good from poor results of saphenous surgery much earlier than was possible formerly.

SAPHENOUS SCLEROTHERAPY

Minimally invasive obliteration of the saphenous vein to remove it from the circulation has been a tantalizing possibility ever since the invention of the syringe in the mid-19th century. Duplex scanning has allowed recent evaluation of this maneuver using relatively high-concentration sclerotherapy. In one study from California, 51 of 89 injected limbs (57%) showed greater saphenous vein reflux at the saphenofemoral junction. Reflux down the more distal greater saphenous vein was found in 67 of 89 injected limbs (75%).[8]

Although advocates of sclerotherapy in general, and duplex-guided sclerotherapy in particular, objected to the conclusions of that report,[14] an important conclusion was drawn from that study which carries over into present practice. That conclusion was summarized in a letter to the editor of the *Journal of Vascular Surgery*:

> ...(I) fully concur with the conclusion of the authors, namely, that in the presence of hemodynamically significant reflux originating at the level of an incompetent saphenofemoral junction, sclerotherapy treatment of the greater saphenous vein and its varicose tributaries will be short-lived.[15]

Duplex-guided sclerotherapy continues to be practiced even into the 21st century,[16-18] but long-term studies have failed to prove that it is advantageous as compared with high ligation alone, high ligation with sclerotherapy, or sclerotherapy alone. More recent attempts to place the sclerosant solution through an IV catheter have been reported.[19] This maneuver adds interventional radiologists to the listing of persons who care for venous disorders. This technique mirrors experience obtained in the 1950s when surgical placement of the catheter and injection of sclerosant were practiced with disastrous results.[20,21]

A 10-year report comparing endovascular saphenous sclerotherapy with surgical ligation of the saphenofemoral junction and surgical ligation of the saphenofemoral junction plus sclerotherapy has demonstrated the superior results of surgery and the inferior results of sclerotherapy.[22] Even though sclerotherapy failed to control saphenofemoral junction incompetence in 18.8% of cases and failed to obliterate distal saphenous reflux in 43.8% of cases, the conclusion of this report was that endovascular sclerotherapy is an effective, cheaper treatment option.[22]

HISTORIC ATTEMPTS AT SAPHENOUS ABLATION

Attempts to destroy vascular walls by coagulation have a long history. Initial attempts involved creation of a thrombus within the vessel lumen. One method was to apply direct current to the outside of the vessel wall.[23] In theory, the negative charge on platelets would be attracted to the positive charge on the electrode on the vessel wall, and the resulting platelet aggregation would initiate the coagulation cascade. This theory was supported by studies that demonstrated that the amount of thrombus formed by direct-current application to the splenic artery was less in volume in thrombocytopenic animals.[24] Direct-current application to the adventitia of vessels produced occlusion but only after several hours of stimulation. It was logical, therefore, to shift to an intraluminal supply of direct current.[25] As this was done, a shift to alternating current was also achieved.[26] Thus, thrombotic occlusion time was reduced to a matter of 10 to 20 seconds.

In general, direct and alternating currents produce vessel occlusion in different ways. Direct current causes localized thrombosis by prolonged electrolysis. In contrast, high-frequency alternating current causes a rapid thermic electrocoagulation. Prolonged exposure to high-frequency alternating current results in total loss of vessel wall architecture, disintegration, and carbonization.[27] Application of this knowledge allowed treatment of the greater saphenous vein by intraluminal techniques.[28] The "excellent" results obtained in 389 patients were clouded by third-degree burns of the skin, saphenous nerve injury, periphlebitis, peroneal nerve injury, and wound infection.[29] Thus, the need for careful monitoring of injury parameters was recognized.

ELECTROMAGNETIC THERAPY

New instrumentation has been devised to deal with both aspects of the surgical treatment of varicose veins. Elimination of saphenous vein reflux has been accomplished by using radiofrequency heating (Fig 1).[30] The VNUS vein treatment system using the Closure catheter (VNUS Medical Technologies, Sunnyvale, Calif) is the most frequently used system in this country and in Western Europe. This system uses electrodes specifically designed for treat-

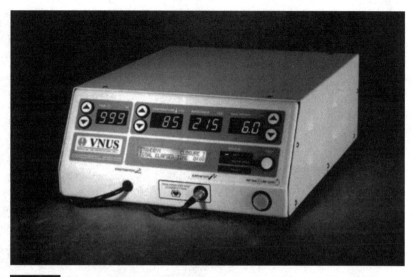

FIGURE 1.

The radiofrequency generator is shown here. The displays from **left** to **right** are radiofrequency generation time, temperature as registered by the thermocouple, impedance, and power in watts. In practice, the temperature becomes the dominant control and is kept as close to 85°C as possible.

ment of the saphenous vein and includes monitoring of electrical and thermal effects of the catheter (Fig 2). Clinically, the device produces precise tissue destruction with minimal formation of thrombus. Bipolar electrodes are used to heat the vein wall. The net effect is venous spasm and collagen shrinkage that produce maximal physical contraction (Fig 3).

In practice, elimination of venous flow is accomplished by Esmarch bandaging and proximal saphenofemoral junction compression. Saphenous vein ablation has been performed using IV sedation and tumescent anesthesia alone[31] and with general anesthesia,[32] with and without proximal saphenofemoral ligation.[33] Acute closure has been achieved in 93% of 141 saphenous veins in the first large series to be reported,[34] and 1-year continued closure exceeds 90%, with only a small fraction of the original anatomical failures requiring re-treatment.[35]

Surgical series have shown that undesirable outcomes after saphenous stripping are evident early.[9] It is acknowledged that surgical stripping results in recurrent truncal vein reflux in 20% of limbs[12] and that 73% of limbs destined for recurrent varicosities at 5 years have already done so at 1 year.[13] Thus, the 1-year results of VNUS

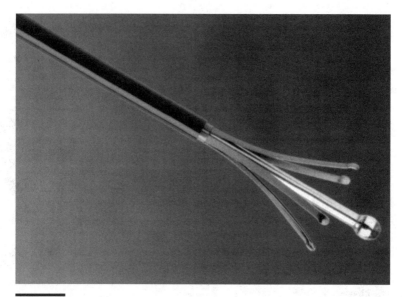

FIGURE 2.
The 6F catheter supplements the previously issued 5F and 8F catheters, and the thermocouple is shown on the **right**.

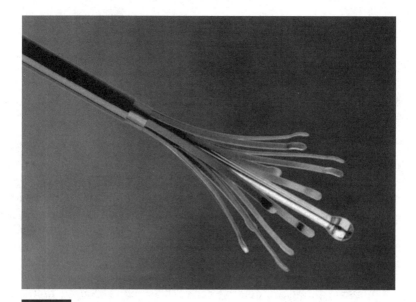

FIGURE 3.
The 8F catheter is shown fully opened to emphasize the rounded tip, which allows easy passage of the catheter in the saphenous vein.

Closure seem destined to be comparable to stripping in the long term.

Goldman,[36] who has taken the lead in endovenous closure in our office, uses large amounts of tumescent anesthesia containing 0.1% lidocaine with epinephrine. Intraoperative ultrasound monitoring ensures that the greater saphenous vein is separated from the skin by the tumescent anesthesia, thus avoiding skin burns.

Performing endovenous obliteration of the saphenous vein without dissection of the saphenofemoral junction violates a cardinal rule in saphenous vein surgery, namely that each of the tributaries must be individually divided. Some investigators advocate that each of the tributaries should be dissected back beyond their primary and even secondary tributaries.[37]

Careful duplex evaluation of saphenous obliteration by Pichot et al[38] has revealed marked shrinking and obliteration of the saphenous vein itself but with preservation of tributaries to the saphenofemoral junction. A discussion of this finding occurred at the annual meeting of the American Venous Forum in February 2000.[39] Sixty limbs treated with saphenofemoral junction ligation and division of tributaries were compared with 120 limbs treated without high ligation. Of the 49 high-ligation limbs followed up for a sufficient length of time, 2% developed recurrent reflux by 6 months, whereas in the 97 limbs treated without high ligation followed up for that length of time, 8% developed recurrent reflux (P = NS). In limbs followed up to 12 months, no new instances of reflux developed. Actuarial recurrence curves were not different with or without saphenofemoral ligation, and the experience predicted a greater than 90% freedom from recurrent reflux and varicosities at 1 year for both groups.

The issue is not settled, but it is acknowledged that should a tributary develop reflux and prove to be a source of recurrent varicosities, the problem can be managed without further surgery by using sclerotherapy. Many surgeons would prefer ambulatory phlebectomy at this point, but in either event, the problem is not a major deterrent to use of endovascular saphenous vein obliteration by radiofrequency energy without saphenofemoral ligation.

CONCLUSIONS

Removal of the saphenous vein from the circulation is a primary part of varicose vein surgery and can be achieved by physical removal or simple destruction. Use of radiofrequency energy allows total coagulation of vein proteins and produces rapid total destruction of the treated vein. This technique is associated with a considerable decrease in postoperative discomfort.

REFERENCES

1. Callam MJ: Epidemiology of varicose veins. *Br J Surg* 81:167-173, 1994.
2. Bergan JJ: A unifying concept of primary venous insufficiency. *Dermatol Surg* 24:425-428, 1998.
3. Cotton LT: Varicose veins: Gross anatomy and development. *Br J Surg* 48:589-598, 1961.
4. Walsh JC, Bergan JJ, Beeman S, et al: Femoral venous reflux abolished by greater saphenous vein stripping. *Ann Vasc Surg* 8:566-570, 1994.
5. Padberg FT, Pappas PJ, Araki CT, et al: Hemodynamic and clinical improvement after superficial vein ablation in primary combined venous insufficiency with ulceration. *J Vasc Surg* 24:711-719, 1996.
6. Neglen P, Einarsson E, Eklof B: The functional long- term value of different types of treatment for saphenous vein incompetence. *J Cardiovasc Surg* 34:295-301, 1993.
7. Goren G, Yellin AE: Minimally invasive surgery for primary varicose veins: Limited invaginated axial stripping and tributary (hook) stab avulsion. *Ann Vasc Surg* 9:401-414, 1995.
8. Bishop CC, Fronek HS, Fronek A, et al: Real-time color duplex scanning after sclerotherapy of the greater saphenous vein. *J Vasc Surg* 14:505-510, 1991.
9. Sarin S, Scurr JH, Coleridge Smith PD: Assessment of stripping the long saphenous vein in the treatment of primary varicose veins. *Br J Surg* 79:889-893, 1992.
10. Rutgers PH, Kistlaar PJEHM: Randomized trial of stripping versus high ligation combined with sclerotherapy in the treatment of the incompetent greater saphenous vein. *Am J Surg* 168:311-315, 1994.
11. Nyamekye I, Shephard NA, Davies B, et al: Clinicopathological evidence that neovascularization is a cause of recurrent varicose veins. *Eur J Vasc Endovasc Surg* 15:412-415, 1998.
12. Dwerryhouse S, Davies B, Harradine K, et al: Stripping the long saphenous vein reduces the rate of reoperation for recurrent varicose veins: Five-year results of a randomized trial. *J Vasc Surg* 29:589-592, 1999.
13. Jones L, Braithwaite BD, Selwyn D, et al: Neovascularization is the principal cause of varicose vein recurrence: Results of a randomized trial of stripping the long saphenous vein. *Eur J Vasc Endovasc Surg* 12:442-445, 1996.
14. Isaacs N: Letter to the editor. *J Vasc Surg* 16:497-498, 1992.
15. Goren G: Letter to the editor. *J Vasc Surg* 16:497-498, 1992.
16. Cornu-Thenard A, de Cottreau H, Weiss RA: Sclerotherapy: Continuous-wave Doppler-guided injections. *Dermatol Surg* 21:867-870, 1995.
17. Kanter A: Clinical determinants of ultrasound-guided sclerotherapy

outcome. Part I: The effects of age, gender, and vein size. *Dermatol Surg* 24:131-135, 1998.

18. Kanter A: Clinical determinants of ultrasound-guided sclerotherapy outcome. Part II: The search of the ideal injectate volume. *Dermatol Surg* 24:136-140, 1998.

19. Min RJ, Navarro L: Transcatheter duplex ultrasound-guided sclerotherapy for treatment of greater saphenous vein reflux: A preliminary report. *Dermatol Surg* 26:410-414, 2000.

20. DePalma RG, Rose SS, Bergan JJ: Treatment of varicosities of saphenous origin: A dialogue, in Goldman MP, Weiss RA, Bergan JJ (eds): *Varicose Veins & Telangiectasias: Diagnosis and Management*, ed 2. St Louis, Quality Medical Publishing, 1999, pp 193-225.

21. McPheeters HO: Saphenofemoral ligation with the immediate retrograde injection. *Surg Gynecol Obstet* 81:355-364, 1945.

22. Belcaro G, Nicolaides AN, Ricci A, et al: Endovascular sclerotherapy, surgery, and surgery plus sclerotherapy for superficial venous incompetence: A randomized 10-year followup trial: Final results. *Angiology* 51:529-534, 2000.

23. Sawyer PN, Page JW: Bioelectric phenomena as an etiologic factor in intravascular thrombosis. *Am J Physiol* 175:103-107, 1953.

24. Thompson WM, Pizzo S, Jackson DC, et al: The effect of drug-induced thrombocytopenia on direct-current transcatheter electrocoagulation. *Works in Progress* 124:831-833, 1977.

25. Phillips JF, Robinson AE, Johnsrude IS, et al: Experimental closure of arteriovenous fistula by transcatheter electrocoagulation. *Radiology* 115:319-321, 1975.

26. Brunelle F, Kunstlinger F, Quillard J: Endovascular electrocoagulation with a bipolar electrode and alternating current: A followup study in dogs. *Radiology* 148:413-415, 1993.

27. Sigel B, Dunn MR: The mechanism of blood vessel closure by high-frequency electrocoagulation. *Surg Gynecol Obstet* 823-831, 1965.

28. Politowski M, Szpak E, Marszalek Z: Varices of the lower extremities treated by electrocoagulation. *Surgery* 66:355-360, 1964.

29. Politowski M, Zelazny T: Complications and difficulties in electrocoagulation of varices of the lower extremities. *Surgery* 59:932-934, 1966.

30. Weiss RA, Goldman MP: Controlled RF-mediated endovenous shrinkage and occlusion, in Goldman MP, Weiss RA, Bergan JJ (eds): *Varicose Veins & Telangiectasias: Diagnosis and Management*, ed 3. St Louis, Quality Medical Publishing, 289-293, 1999.

31. Goldman MP: Closure of the greater saphenous vein with endoluminal radiofrequency thermal heating of the vein wall in combination with ambulatory phlebectomy: Preliminary 6-month followup. *Dermatol Surg* 26:105, 2000.

32. Chandler JG, Pichot O, Sessa C, et al: Treatment of primary venous insufficiency by endovenous saphenous vein obliteration. *Vasc Surg* 34:201-214, 2000.

33. Whiteley MS, Pichot O, Sessa C, et al: Endovenous obliteration: An effective, minimally invasive surrogate for saphenous vein stripping. *J Endovasc Surg* 7:I1-I7, 2000.

34. Manfrini S, Gasbarro V, Danielsson G, et al: Endovenous management of saphenous vein reflux. *J Vasc Surg* 32:330-342, 2000.

35. Chandler JG: Personal communication.

36. Goldman MP: Closure of the greater saphenous vein with endoluminal radiofrequency thermal heating of the vein wall in combination with ambulatory phlebectomy: Preliminary 6-month followup. *Dermatol Surg* 26:452-456, 2000.

37. Bergan JJ: Saphenous vein stripping by inversion: Current technique. *Surg Rounds* 34:118-124, 2000.

38. Pichot O, Sessa C, Chandler JG, et al: Role of duplex imaging in endovenous obliteration for primary venous insufficiency. *J Endovasc Ther* 7:451-459, 2000.

39. Chandler JG, Pichot O, Sessa C, et al: Defining the role of extended saphenofemoral junction ligation: A prospective comparative study. *J Vasc Surg* 32:941-953, 2000.

CHAPTER 10

Management of Deep Vein Thrombosis in Pregnancy

Sonia S. Anand, MD, MSc
Assistant Professor of Medicine, Department of Medicine, McMaster
University, and Vascular Medicine Specialist, Hamilton Health Sciences
Corporation, Hamilton, Ontario, Canada

Samuel Z. Goldhaber, MD
Associate Professor of Medicine, Harvard Medical School, and Director,
Venous Thromboembolism Research Group, Brigham and Women's
Hospital, Boston, Mass

Venous thromboembolism in pregnancy is an important cause of maternal death. Pregnancy is considered to be a "risk factor" for deep vein thrombosis (DVT) because the risk of venous thromboembolism is five times higher in pregnant women compared with nonpregnant women of similar age.[1] The increased incidence of DVT in pregnancy likely reflects the increased venous stasis and the hypercoaguable state of pregnancy, which is characterized by increases in procoagulant factors such as fibrinogen, factor VIII, and factor V, as well as impairment of the fibrinolytic process.[1,2]

EPIDEMIOLOGY OF THROMBOSIS IN PREGNANCY

Although the true incidence of DVT in pregnancy is unknown, the incidence of venous thromboembolism is approximately 1 per 1000.[1] The incidence of DVT is the highest among pregnant women who are older, overweight, who have abnormal levels of coagulation factors that increase the chance of thrombosis (thrombophilia), and who have had a prior DVT.[2,3] DVT can occur in any stage of pregnancy, with almost 50% of all DVTs being diagnosed in the first and second trimesters.[4] The postpartum state, which is defined as the period between delivery and 6 weeks after delivery, also represents a high-risk state, and the incidence of DVT is approximately 0.5 per 1000.[2] Furthermore, there is a strong predilection for DVTs to occur in the left leg, most likely because of compression of the left iliac vein by the right iliac and ovarian arteries as they cross over it.[2,5]

DIAGNOSIS OF DVT IN PREGNANCY

In pregnant patients with DVT or pulmonary embolism, accurate diagnosis is required to identify patients who require anticoagulant therapy, and to reliably exclude DVT among patients without this illness so they are not exposed to the risks of anticoagulants.[6] The diagnosis of DVT in pregnancy is made by combining the clinical probability (based on the history and physical examination) with the results of objective diagnostic tests. The essential features of the clinical assessment include a comprehensive history and physical examination. Although no formal scoring system to generate the pretest probability of thrombosis has been validated in pregnant women, given the increased risk of thrombosis in pregnancy, women who have symptoms of unilateral leg pain or swelling should receive a thorough workup for DVT.

BIOCHEMICAL MARKERS

D-dimer is a fibrin degradation product that is associated with the breakdown of thrombus. Levels are often measured in patients with suspected venous thromboembolism before diagnostic imaging. Normal values of D-dimer are strongly associated with the absence of venous thromboembolism in the nonpregnant state. Recent data indicate that D-dimer levels gradually increase over time in uncomplicated pregnancies.[7,8] However, the diagnostic value of D-dimer levels in pregnancy has not been well evaluated, and therefore it is not recommended that D-dimer levels be used to assist in the diagnosis of DVT in pregnancy.

IMAGING MODALITIES

The standard diagnostic test used to detect DVT in the lower extremities in pregnant women is duplex compression ultrasound (CUS).[9] In nonpregnant patients, the sensitivity and specificity of CUS are high, making it an excellent first option. The finding of a noncompressible venous segment has a high positive predictive value for DVT (Fig 1). However, pregnant women are at increased risk of having iliac vein thrombosis, which is not adequately assessed by duplex CUS.[2,6] A decreased Doppler flow signal in the common femoral vein suggests that a more proximal venous obstruction exists either extrinsic to the pelvic vessels (ie, secondary to an enlarged uterus) or intrinsic, caused by thrombosis (Fig 2). However, a normal Doppler flow signal in the common

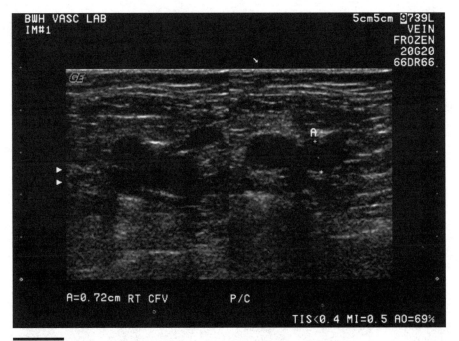

FIGURE 1.
White arrows denote the precompression view of the right superficial femoral and profunda arteries adjacent to the right common femoral vein *(RT CFV)*. The RT CFV fails to compress (denoted by the letter *A*) in the partial compression image. This is diagnostic of deep vein thrombosis.

femoral vein does not rule out the presence of a more proximal thrombosis. Thus, in pregnant patients who have reduced flow in the common femoral vein seen with Doppler, or in whom iliac vein thrombosis is strongly suspected, additional diagnostic testing is required. Depending on the availability of imaging, either ascending venography or magnetic resonance (MR) imaging can be used. When venography is performed, a persistent intraluminal filling defect present in at least two views is diagnostic of DVT.[1] A diagnosis of venous thrombosis is possible with fetal radiation exposure of less than .005 Gy when venography is performed when the patient's abdomen is shielded. This is significantly less than the doses of in utero radiation that are associated with childhood cancers (ie, .05 Gy or greater), and significantly less than that of a standard chest radiograph.[10] The advantages of MR angiography over venography include avoidance of iodinated contrast and radiation exposure (Fig 3).[1,11]

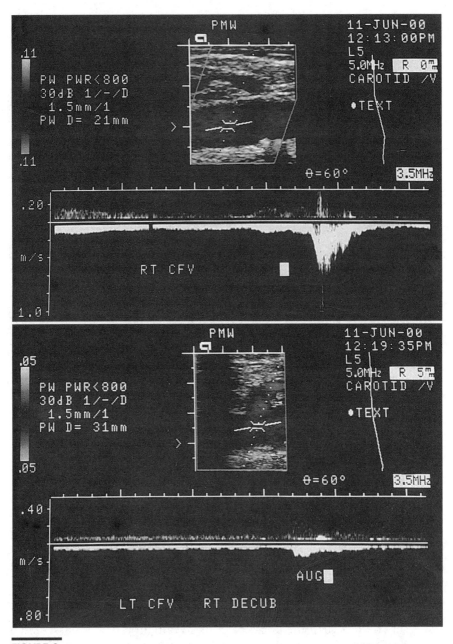

FIGURE 2.
Absence of respiratory variation in the Doppler signal is noted on the left common femoral vein *(LT CFV)* tracing compared with the right common femoral vein *(RT CFV)* tracing. This is suggestive of a more proximal venous compression.

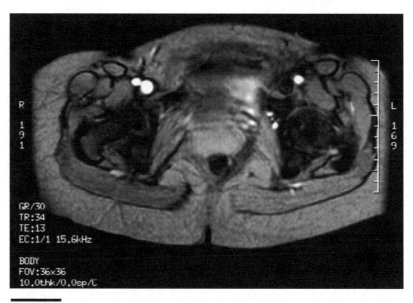

FIGURE 3.
Magnetic resonance imaging using bright blood GRASS (gradient-recalled acquisition in the steady-state) images demonstrates normal iliac venous and arterial filling of the right pelvic vessels, and absence of venous filling of the left iliac vein, which is diagnostic of acute thrombosis.

TREATMENT OF DVT IN PREGNANCY
RATIONALE FOR TREATMENT

DVT in pregnancy requires treatment with systemic doses of anticoagulants because of the potential risk of pulmonary embolus to the mother, which jeopardizes the well-being of the fetus. Full-dose anticoagulation should be initiated regardless of the stage of pregnancy, and continued throughout the pregnancy and postpartum state (6 weeks after delivery).[1,6] Alternatives, such as observation with serial ultrasound testing, use of prophylactic doses of anticoagulants, and/or aspirin therapy in place of full-dose anticoagulation, are unacceptable and potentially life-threatening.

CHOICE OF ANTICOAGULANT

Anticoagulation in pregnancy is challenging because oral anticoagulants can cause embryopathy, and heparins, although they do not cross the placenta, can cause bleeding and osteoporosis.[6] Systemic anticoagulation for DVT in pregnancy may be attained by using unfractionated heparin (UFH) or low–molecular weight heparin (LMWH).[6] Oral anticoagulants, such as warfarin, are generally not accepted for use in pregnancy in the United States. Neither UFH nor LMWH crosses the placenta, and neither is fetopathic. LMWH is becoming more popular than UFH in the treatment of DVT.

MONITORING ANTICOAGULANTS

UFH is traditionally monitored by using the activated partial thromboplastin time (aPTT), which is sensitive to the inhibition of thrombin, factor Xa, and factor IXa.[12] The therapeutic range for UFH using the aPTT differs for different reagents, and a fixed ratio of 1.5 to 2.5 times control is therapeutic for most reagents. The therapeutic range using the aPTT should correspond to a heparin level of 0.2 to 0.4 U/mL by protamine sulfate titration, or 0.4 to 0.7 U/mL by antifactor Xa assay.[12] Unlike UFH, routine monitoring of LMWH is usually not necessary. However, in certain clinical scenarios, such as renal failure, obesity, and pregnancy, monitoring may be justified.[12] The optimal time to perform the antifactor Xa assay is 3 to 6 hours after a weighted-adjusted dose of LMWH has been given. The therapeutic range for LMWH is approximately 0.5 to 1.0 U/mL, 3 to 6 hours after the subcutaneous injection.[12]

UFH

Administration of UFH has been the traditional approach for treatment of DVT in pregnancy, usually with UFH being given as an IV infusion to target an aPTT of between 1.5 and 2.5 times control.[1,6] Pregnancy is associated with increased heparin-binding proteins, which cause heparin resistance, and therefore increased doses of UFH are usually required for aPTT values to reach therapeutic levels.[13] Once therapeutic levels have been reached, in the face of improving symptoms and the desire to have the patient treated as an outpatient, IV UFH may be switched to the twice-daily UFH subcutaneous injections. It is generally recommended that subcutaneous heparin be given every 12 hours, and monitored by 6-hour postinjection aPTTs or heparin levels to target a range of between 0.4 and 0.7 U/mL using anti–factor Xa levels.[6] For many aPTT reagents, this is equivalent to a ratio (patient/control aPTT) of 1.5 to 2.5. Of note is that the aPTT response in pregnancy is attenuated because factor VIII and fibrinogen levels are increased,[2] and the aPTT values may not directly reflect the anticoagulant state of the patient. Therefore, regular use of heparin levels to monitor patients receiving long-term UFH therapy in pregnancy may be helpful.

LMWHs

LMWHs have been evaluated in a large number of randomized clinical trials and have been shown to be safe and effective for the prevention and treatment of venous thrombosis, acute pulmonary embolism, and for acute coronary syndromes.[12] Although there have been few detailed assessments of LMWH in pregnancy, the clinical experience thus far indicates that LMWH is at least as effective as UFH.[14,15] Furthermore, there are other advantages of LMWH over UFH, such as a more predictable dose response, ease of administration, lower incidence of heparin-induced thrombocytopenia, and less osteopenia.[6,15] Two LMWH preparations have been used in pregnancy: enoxaparin, given subcutaneously in a dosage of 1 mg/kg every 12 hours, or as a single injection of 1.5 mg/kg per day; and dalteparin, given subcutaneously in a dosage of either 100 U/kg twice a day, or 200 U/kg once per day.[6] Routine monitoring of the LMWH is not required, unless the patient develops bleeding, recurrent venous thromboembolism, is obese, or has renal insufficiency. However, to gain clinical experience with LMWH in pregnancy, some clinicians choose to monitor anti–factor Xa heparin levels 3 to 6 hours after the morning dose to target an anti–factor Xa level of between 0.6 and 1.0 U/mL.[6]

INTRACAVAL FILTERS

Intracaval filters have been used in selected cases of venous thromboembolism during pregnancy; however, the clinical experience with these devices is limited. Concerns about location of placement as well as radiation exposure to the fetus are warranted. Currently, the use of caval filters should be reserved for pregnant patients who have recurrence of venous thrombosis despite systemic anticoagulation, and for patients who cannot receive anticoagulation with UFH or LMWH because of bleeding.

MANAGEMENT OF ANTICOAGULATION AT THE TIME OF DELIVERY

Because of the expected bleeding associated with delivery, the management of pregnant patients with DVT must be altered before delivery. Ideally, approximately 24 hours before delivery, full-dose anticoagulation is held, and then reintroduced after delivery when the bleeding risk of the mother has been reduced.[6] However, because the onset of labor is not a predictable event, two standard approaches are recommended. First, for the patient who wishes a trial of natural labor and delivery, the twice-daily injections of UFH or LMWH should be switched 3 weeks before the due date to UFH injections three times per day to target a 4-hour postinjection aPTT of between 1.5 and 2.5 times control or an anti–factor Xa level of 0.4 to 0.7 U/mL. Heparin is then withheld at the onset of labor. There appears to be a persistent anticoagulant effect with UFH for up to 28 hours after the last injection. Therefore, the aPTT should be checked before epidural placement or delivery, and if prolonged, protamine should be given to normalize the aPTT, to decrease the risk of epidural hematoma and bleeding.[6] Second, if a cesarean section is planned, the twice-daily UFH or LMWH injections should be stopped 24 hours before surgery, and an aPTT (in the case of UFH) or an anti–factor Xa heparin level (in the case of LMWH) should be drawn before epidural placement to ensure that the heparin effect has been reversed. In certain high-risk cases, after the subcutaneous injections are stopped, IV UFH may be given to ensure that the patient is covered for as long as possible before delivery.

MANAGEMENT OF ANTICOAGULATION AFTER DELIVERY

After delivery, in general, all women in whom a DVT was diagnosed during their pregnancy should continue to receive systemic antico-agulant therapy for at least 6 weeks.[2,6] Options include continuing injections of full-dose UFH or LMWH, or use of LMWH as a bridge to warfarin to target an international normalized ratio of 2 to 3. Nursing mothers of the offspring should be advised that neither heparin nor warfarin appears to affect the coagulation status.[2,6] It should be noted that the postpartum period is also a high-risk state for venous thromboembolism, and since the 1980s, the incidence of DVT in the postpartum state after cesarean section and vaginal delivery has increased.[2] Therefore, thromboprophylaxis should be considered on a case-by-case basis after delivery in all women.

ADJUNCTIVE TREATMENT

Apart from full-dose anticoagulation, adjunctive treatment strategies for DVT in pregnancy require consideration. First, graded compres-sion stockings, either in the form of above-the-knee panty hose at 20 to 30 mm Hg of pressure, or as below-the-knee stockings at 20 to 40 mm Hg of pressure will reduce leg swelling. Second, many women require additional emotional support to help allay fears about recur-rent thrombosis or bleeding, and the risks that these two events may pose to themselves and to the fetus.

CONCLUSION

DVT in pregnancy is a potentially life-threatening condition. Cli-nicians must be aware of the potential pitfalls in the diagnosis of

DVT, such as normal findings on duplex ultrasound in the presence of iliac vein thrombosis, and must perform more invasive testing when the clinical suspicion of DVT is high. The mainstay of treatment for DVT in pregnancy includes full-dose anticoagulation with either UFH or LMWH. Treatment should continue for at least 6 weeks after delivery.

REFERENCES

1. Toglia MR, Weg JG: Venous thromboembolism during pregnancy. *N Engl J Med* 335:108-114, 1996.
2. Greer IA: Thrombosis in pregnancy: Maternal and fetal issues. *Lancet* 353:1258-1265, 1999.
3. Brill-Edwards P, Ginsberg JS, Gent M, et al: Safety of withholding heparin in pregnant women with a history of venous thromboembolism. *N Engl J Med* 343:1439-1444, 2000.
4. Ray JG, Chan WS: Deep vein thrombosis during pregnancy and the puerperium: A meta-analysis of the period of risk and the leg of presentation. *Obstet Gynecol Surv* 54:265-271, 1999.
5. Ginsberg JS, Brill-Edwards P, Burrows RF, et al: DVT during pregnancy: Leg and trimester of presentation. *Thromb Haemost* 67:519-520, 1992.
6. Ginsberg JS, Greer I, Hirsh J: Use of antithrombotic agents during pregnancy. *Chest* 119:122S-131S, 2001.
7. Comeglio F, Alessandrello L, Cellai L, et al: D-dimer plasma levels during normal pregnancy measured by specific ELISA. *Int J Clin Lab Res* 27:65-67, 1997.
8. Walterman E, Hafner P, Kaider A, et al: Prospective evaluation of hemostatic system activation and thrombin potential in healthy pregnant women with and without factor V Leiden. *Thromb Haemost* 82:1232-1236, 1999.
9. Lensing AWA, Prandoni P, Brandjes D, et al: Detection of deep-vein thrombosis by real time B-mode ultrasonography. *N Engl J Med* 320:342-345, 1989.
10. Ginsberg JS, Hirsh J, Rainbow AJ, et al: Risks to the fetus of radiologic procedures used in the diagnosis of maternal venous thromboembolic disease. *Thromb Haemost* 61:189-196, 1989.
11. Spritzer CE, Evans AC, Kay HH: Magnetic resonance imaging of deep venous thrombosis in pregnant women with lower extremity edema. *Obstet Gynecol* 85:603-607, 1995.
12. Hirsh J, Warkentin T, Shaughnessy S, et al: Heparin and low molecular weight heparin: Mechanisms of action, pharmacokinetics, dosing, monitoring, efficacy, and safety. *Chest* 199:64S-94S, 2001.
13. Anand SS, Brimble S, Ginsberg JS: Management of iliofemoral thrombosis in a pregnant patient with heparin resistance. *Arch Intern Med* 157:815-816, 1997.
14. Chan WS, Ray JG: Low molecular weight heparin use during preg-

nancy: Issues of safety and practicality. *Obstet Gynecol Surv* 54:649-654, 1999.
15. Sanson BJ, Lensing AW, Prins MH, et al: Safety of low-molecular-weight heparin in pregnancy: A systematic review. *Thromb Haemost* 81:668-672, 1999.

CHAPTER 11

Anomalies of Inferior Vena Cava and Left Renal Vein Complicate Traditional Aortic Surgery

Lee Kirksey, MD
Fellow in Vascular Surgery, Newark Beth Israel Medical Center,
St. Barnabas Health Care System, Newark, NJ

Bruce J. Brener, MD
Associate Clinical Professor of Surgery, Columbia University, and Chief,
Vascular Surgery, Newark Beth Israel Medical Center, Newark, NJ

Contemporary series of abdominal aortic aneurysm (AAA) repair report operative mortality rates approaching 3% to 5%.[1,2] A possible contributor to operative mortality is venous hemorrhage. Venous anomalies are relatively uncommon but when they are unrecognized, injury during clamping of the juxtarenal aneurysm neck or iliac arteries may result in hemorrhage, significantly complicating the elective repair of an AAA. We describe the embryologic, anatomic, and radiographic findings associated with these venous anomalies. In addition, we discuss several technical maneuvers that may be helpful in the management of these venous anomalies. Familiarity with the developmental origin, identification, and management of these uncommon anomalies will allow the surgeon to anticipate and manage these problems effectively.

Four major venous anomalies have been identified, described, and encountered during aortic surgery. Two variations involving the inferior vena cava (IVC) include the duplicated IVC and the transposed (left-sided) IVC. Two variations of renal vein anatomy are the retroaortic left renal vein and the circumaortic renal collar. Two other anomalies, caval interruption with azygous connection and retrocaval ureter, are uncommon and will not be discussed.

EMBRYOLOGY

From the sixth through the eighth week of fetal development, the anatomy of the infrahepatic IVC and renal vein changes quickly and dramatically. Three parallel sets of veins appear, connect, and partially recede. These veins, in order of their appearance, are the posterior cardinal, subcardinal, and supracardinal.

The posterior cardinal veins are the most primitive and, after connecting with the subcardinal veins, persist only as the iliac veins and the iliac bifurcation. The right and left subcardinal veins develop anastomoses with each other and lie ventral to the aorta. The right subcardinal vein persists as the suprarenal vena cava. The left subcardinal vein persists as the adrenal vein. The supracardinal veins develop last. They gradually become the primary venous drainage of the caudal part of the body. These vessels, which lie dorsal to the aorta, anastomose with themselves and with the subcardinal veins to form a renal collar. The right supracardinal vein persists as the normal infrarenal segment of the IVC. The renal veins are formed by the anastomosis of the supracardinal and subcardinal veins. Two renal veins form (ventral and dorsal); however, the dorsal vein usually degenerates, and the ventral vein forms the renal vein.[3]

If the left supracardinal vein fails to involute, the vena cava may remain as a duplicated structure. If the right supracardinal vein disappears, but the left remains, a left-sided cava or "transposition" exists. The "circumaortic or periaortic renal ring or collar" may develop if the subcardinal and supracardinal veins fail to involute. In the normal form, the left renal vein remains ventral to the aorta, and the retroaortic component regresses. The dorsal portion of the collar may persist and the ventral vein may involute, resulting in the so-called retroaortic renal vein.

Thus, the anomalies have been classified as follows[4]:

1. Anomalies of the posterior cardinal veins
   - Retrocaval/circumcaval ureter
2. Anomalies of the subcardinal veins
   - Interruption of the IVC with azygous/hemiazygous continuation
3. Anomalies of the supracardinal veins
   - Persistence of the left supracardinal vein-left IVC
   - Persistence of both left and right supracardinal veins-double IVC
4. Anomalies of the renal segment formed by the subcardinal/supracardinal venous anastomoses
   - Circumaortic venous ring
   - Retroaortic renal vein
   - Multiple renal veins

INCIDENCE

Currently, computed tomographic (CT) scan is the imaging modality of choice for the preoperative evaluation of a patient with an AAA. The addition of spiral CT with 3-dimensional reconstruction facilitates a noninvasive assessment of the renal vasculature with better resolution than was previously possible with catheter arteriography.

The incidence of venous anomalies as reported in the anatomic and surgical literature is listed in Table 1.[5] The left-sided IVC is a rare anomaly and is radiographically obvious and easily identified at operation (Fig 1). In contrast, the left portion of the double cava may be small and easily overlooked during dissection. The double IVC has a reported incidence of 2% to 3% in autopsy series.[6] In studies using CT scan, the incidence was only 0.3%, suggesting that the smaller left component may not be seen on CT imaging. Misdiagnosis of the aberrant left IVC as lymphadenopathy should be avoided.

A circumaortic renal collar is relatively common, with a reported incidence of 1.5% to 8.7%.[7] In analysis of 433 CT scans, this anomaly was identified in 19 cases (4.4%).[8] The incidence of renal collar may be as high as 16% if all retroaortic venous structures are considered. At surgery, it is common to see large venous structures to the left of the aorta communicating with the lumbar veins, the left renal vein, and the IVC. In fact, in autopsy series, the incidence of circumaortic renal collar was 16.8%, again suggesting that preoperative CT scanning is not sensitive (Fig 2).[9] The retroaortic renal vein has been noted in about 2% of patients.[5]

RECOGNITION

The importance of intraoperative recognition cannot be overemphasized. Anomalous venous anatomy presents a threat of serious hemorrhage if unsuspected, especially if circumferential dissection of the aorta and iliac arteries is habitually employed.

TABLE 1.

Incidence of Previously Described Venous Anomalies

Anomaly	Incidence (%)
Left IVC	0.2-0.5
Double IVC	2.2-3.0
Circumaortic renal collar	1.5-8.7
Retroaortic left renal vein	1.8-2.4

Abbreviation: IVC, Inferior vena cava.

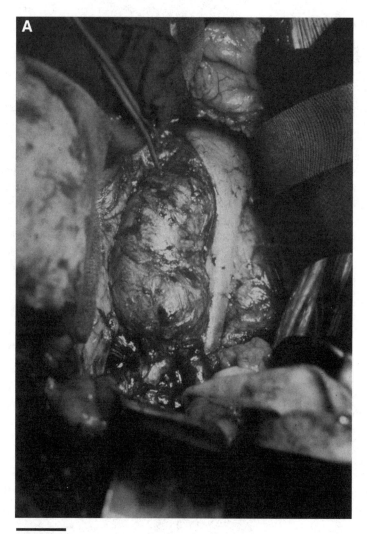

FIGURE 1.
A, Intraoperative photograph of left-sided inferior vena cava (IVC).

(continued)

In contrast to the 1970s when injury to the venous structures was not uncommon, accurate preoperative imaging is now the rule rather than the exception. CT is almost always obtained before elective, and often before emergent, aortic surgery. Modern spiral CT images can be rapidly obtained to avoid artifact and reveal all the pertinent venous anomalies. Selective catheterization and direct intravenous contrast to visualize venous anatomy is rarely under-

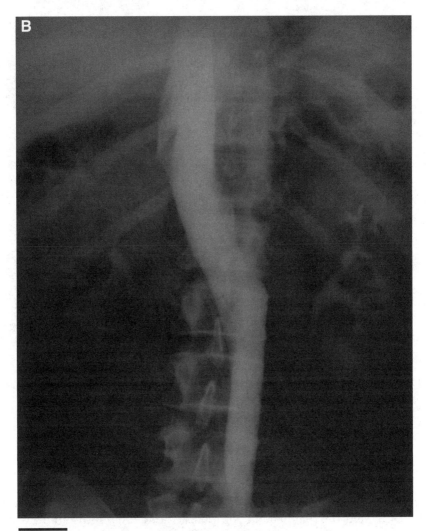

FIGURE 1. (continued)
B, Venography showing left-sided IVC.

taken and is, in general, unnecessary. However, the vascular surgeon may perform direct catheterization during renal vein sampling or vena cava filter placement.

MANAGEMENT
It is axiomatic to state that the newest modality in vascular surgery, endovascular treatment of aortic disease, minimizes the sig-

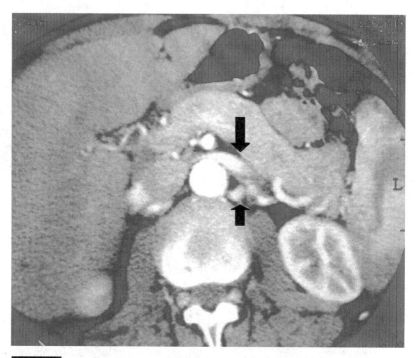

FIGURE 2.
CT image of circumaortic venous collar. The retroaortic portion inserts into
the vena cava more caudally. Larger arrow *(top)* points to the normal ven-
trally located left renal vein. Smaller arrow *(bottom)* indicates retroaortic
portion of left renal vein.

nificance of anomalous venous anatomy. When open reconstruction is planned, careful radiographic evaluation with spiral CT
with 3-dimensional reconstruction permits the preoperative recognition of these findings. Any deviation of normal renal development (ie, renal ectopia or renal fusion) should raise the suspicion
of associated vascular anomalies. An appropriate plan can then be
developed to optimize the management.

As with any operative strategy, the choice of incision is of paramount importance. The retroperitoneal approach through a trans-
verse left flank incision may be problematic if a left-sided cava or
caval duplication is present. Likewise, a retroaortic left renal vein
should be handled carefully if this approach is used.

The retroaortic left renal vein and the renal vein collar will be the
most frequently encountered anomalies noted during the transperi-
toneal dissection of the aorta (Fig 3). Classic teaching suggests that
one should suspect the retroaortic left renal vein when the left renal

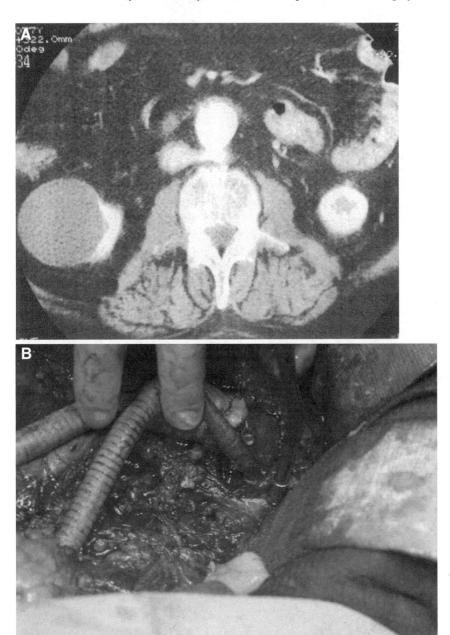

FIGURE 3.
A, Computed tomography (CT) image of retroaortic left renal vein. **B,** Intraoperative photograph of retroaortic renal vein.

vein, normally located anteriorly, is absent or attenuated in size. If a retroaortic venous anomaly is identified, control of the aorta should be obtained above this area. More dangerous is the circumaortic venous collar. In this anomaly, the superior renal vein receives the left adrenal vein and crosses the aorta anteriorly. The inferior renal vein receives the left gonadal vein. Because this occurs in the presence of the normal anterior left renal vein, no clue for identification is present. The single most important fact to be noted is as follows: the insertion of the retroaortic vein into the vena cava in both conditions is usually several centimeters below the normal anterior insertion. Therefore, it is subject to injury if circumaortic dissection is undertaken. Crawford et al[10] showed that the greatest decrease in the mortality rate after AAA repair came with the abandonment of aneurysmectomy in favor of a transluminal repair. Thus, the best way to minimize the possibility of venous injury is to avoid complete circumferential dissection of the aorta and iliac arteries. If dissection is undertaken, it is usually possible to avoid injury through a combination of direct and complete visualization and dissection superior to the vein, immediately below the renal arteries. Injury to the retroaortic vein is no picnic. If direct suture repair is not possible because of inadequate exposure, division of the aorta may be helpful.

The duplicated IVC usually does not provide a major challenge to providing adequate exposure. In this anomaly, the left cava is usually smaller and can be divided safely if necessary (Fig 4). The left renal vein often communicates with the left cava; the renal vein can be divided anteriorly and will drain into the left cava if the latter has not been injured.

The left-sided IVC may provide some serious challenges because it crosses over or under the aorta at the level of the left renal vein. This venous structure may be stretched out and closely applied to the left lateral wall of the aorta. Either division of the cava itself or the right renal vein (medial to its tributaries) has been used to manage this anomaly. The right renal vein is longer and has the same drainage via the adrenal and genital veins that one would expect from a normal left renal vein.

CONCLUSION

Anomalies of the infrahepatic venous circulation have been well described during the last 20 years. The preoperative recognition of these anomalies, by the use of spiral CT scans, has facilitated operative planning. Despite anticipation of these findings, operative injury remains possible, particularly under the circumstances of emergent AAA reconstruction. The vascular surgeon should be

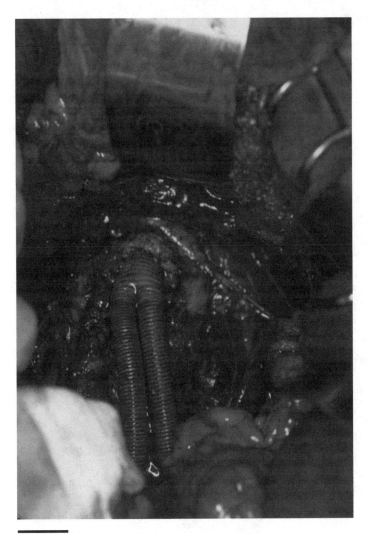

FIGURE 4.
Intraoperative photograph of duplicated inferior vena cava.

familiar with the technical maneuvers that allow the safe management of these venous anomalies. In general, limitation of circumaortic mobilization and careful dissection, combined with the recognition of the location of these vessels, will usually prevent serious life-threatening injuries. Lastly, in the setting of complex venous anomalies, thoughtful consideration should be given to the endovascular method of AAA repair.

REFERENCES

1. Lawrence PF, Gazak C, Bhirangi L, et al: The epidemiology of surgically repaired aneurysms in the United States. *J Vasc Surg* 30:632-640, 1999.
2. Lloyd WE, Paty PS, Darling RC III, et al: Results of 1000 consecutive elective abdominal aortic aneurysm repairs. *Cardiovasc Surg* 4:724-726, 1996.
3. Anson BJ, Cauldwell EW, Pick JW, et al: The anatomy of the pararenal system of veins with comments on the renal arteries. *J Urol* 60:714-737, 1948.
4. Mathews R, Smith P, Fishman EK, et al: Anomalies of the inferior vena cava and renal veins: Embryologic and surgical considerations. *Urology* 53:873-880, 1999.
5. Brener BJ, Darling C, Fredrick PL, et al: Major venous anomalies complicating abdominal aortic surgery. *Arch Surg* 108:160-165, 1974.
6. Baldridge ED Jr, Canos AJ: Venous anomalies encountered in aortoiliac surgery. *Arch Surg* 122:1184-1188, 1987.
7. Giordano JM, Trout HH III: Anomalies of the inferior vena cava. *J Vasc Surg* 3:924-928, 1986.
8. Reed MD, Friedman AC, Neallly P: Anomalies of the left renal vein: Analysis of 433 CT scans. *J Comput Assist Tomogr* 6:1124-1126, 1982.
9. Mayo J, Gray R, Louis ES, et al: Anomalies of the inferior vena cava. *AJR* 140:339-345, 1983.
10. Crawford ES, Saleh SA, Babb JW, et al: Infrarenal abdominal aortic aneurysm: Factors influencing survival after operation performed over a 25 year period. *Ann Surg* 196:699-709, 1981.

PART VI

Issues

CHAPTER 12

Credentialing for Endovascular Techniques

Rodney A. White, MD
Professor of Surgery, University of California at Los Angeles School of
Medicine; Chief, Vascular Surgery, Associate Chairman, Department of
Surgery, Harbor-UCLA Medical Center, Torrance, Calif

Training and credentialing for endovascular procedures is an evolving process as the technologies mature and as various interventional subspecialties adapt training programs to address pertinent issues. Although the ideal would be for institutions to form endovascular services with significant forethought and planning, in most cases, they evolve based on the expertise of individual clinicians who have an interest in adapting newer methods to treat specific illnesses that occur in the particular patient population. In many cases, this may have occurred as interventional radiologists applied their diagnostic imaging and catheter-based skills to the percutaneous treatment of vascular lesions. In addition, peripheral endovascular methods have been applied by surgeons who maintained their diagnostic radiographic skills and began to use endovascular methods as techniques evolved. Cardiologists also treat peripheral vascular lesions as either a means to improve access via peripheral vessels for cardiac interventions, or they use the methods as a part of a combined peripheral and coronary interventional service.

Each subspecialty has specialized skills that influence the efficacy and safe utility of endovascular methods, with the idealized endovascular specialist being an individual who has an extensive knowledge of both catheter-based interventional methods and surgical techniques. The future vascular specialist may be trained in all of these areas. Many institutions are assessing the need for endovascular training and are evaluating the optimal way to accomplish this goal. In the interim, practicing physicians in various subspecialties will be modifying their practice to accommodate the use of endovascular methods. This entails establishing ways to provide training and facilities for application of the methods in an environment that maximizes involvement of appropriate specialties. The role of individuals will vary from institution to institution depending on the particular expertise of those involved and the institutional capabilities to accommodate to the new methods.

CLINICAL SKILLS AND FACILITIES

Although the organization of the endovascular team will be determined by the expertise and interest of various subspecialties and the quality of interventional facilities, two types of clinical skills are required. Interventional catheter-based manipulation and imaging skills are needed for both diagnostic and therapeutic interventions, whereas surgical skills are required to help determine the indications for endovascular therapy compared with conventional surgical treatment. Surgical expertise is also needed to treat possible complications of endovascular mishaps that may require either emergent or elective surgical correction. A combination of interventional catheter and diagnostic skills might be provided by an appropriately trained vascular or cardiovascular surgeon, although the usual scenario in most settings at the present time is that the endovascular team consists of both interventional radiologists and/or cardiologists and vascular surgeons. Although some institutions have been unable to address the development of a service related to either facility constraints or political controversies among the subspecialties, many hospitals are developing congenial arrangements that fulfill the needs of all involved parties.

Several guidelines have been proposed addressing the credentialing and training for various subspecialists to perform endovascular interventions, and there are many points of agreement regarding the essentials for safe application of the technologies.[1-8] Although there are points of disagreement in these documents, ongoing conversations among the involved interventional groups are resolving the remaining issues and delineating mechanisms for addressing controversial areas and establishing an endovascular service in various types of institutional environments. The essentials of establishing an effective environment are those that stimulate the training, credentialing, and practice for the idealized vascular specialist of the future, and those that provide facilities that accommodate the needs of the endovascular team.

CREDENTIALING GUIDELINES
NATIONAL GUIDELINES

The Joint Commission for Accreditation for Health Care Organization (JCAHO) requires that specific privileges be delineated for each hospital staff member. Each hospital is required to monitor the appropriateness of care provided by physicians and to establish mechanisms to assess new technologies before they can be used clinically. These directives have been accommodated in most instances by establishing departmental guidelines for new physicians, or for physicians using techniques or methods that they have not previously used. For interventional and surgical procedures, this usually entails observation of a specified number of procedures by a proctor and the option for reporting of procedural outcomes both initially and after long-term follow-up, if this is considered appropriate by the hospital credentialing body.

Qualifications required for a physician to perform a procedure are based on skills acquired during residency or fellowship training, a supervised preceptorship and/or approved courses when appropriate. Frequently, expertise in new technologies is developed during initial experimental trials of devices by physicians performing the studies under the auspices of institutional review boards and Food and Drug Administration (FDA) investigational programs. Thus, the means by which physicians obtain appropriate training to use new techniques can follow a number of avenues, from formal training to acquisition of skills during initial animal evaluations and clinical trials.

SPECIALTY GUIDELINES

Endovascular device development and application have been influenced by various specialists, primarily surgeons, radiologists, and cardiologists, in the context of how the methods affect each group's primary patient population. Each specialty has independently arrived at training, credentialing, quality assurance, and educational guidelines for applications solely within their discipline (ie, coronary catheterization, cerebral angiography, etc). Controversy and uncertainty have arisen when guidelines are developed for areas of mutual interest (ie, noncoronary angioplasty, stent placement, and endovascular grafting procedures).

This controversy is further complicated because different patient groups may be treated, different criteria of success may be used, and each specialty emphasizes credentialing criteria based on its tradition and the evolution of the endovascular techniques within its domain. Patients who are asymptomatic (minimal disease), or those with intermittent claudication (moderate disease) or limb-threatening ischemia (severe disease) can all be treated by identical techniques. The short- and long-term success in each of these groups is different. Furthermore, whereas immediate hemodynamic or angiographic success is measured by some, long-term clinical evaluation, patency by duplex scan, or hemodynamic success as measured in a noninvasive vascular laboratory are emphasized by others.

Each specialty has established preliminary criteria for application of these endovascular methods based on their interest and ability to treat a particular segment of the patient population and their tradition of equating expertise with numbers of procedures.[1-8] The emphasis in several of the earlier documents is on credentials for percutaneous transluminal angioplasty (PTA), whereas the vascular surgery perspective has been to address more broadly a large number of methods and techniques being developed. Guidelines for procedures in addition to PTA and stent placement will obviously evolve as technology advances and as safety and effectiveness are proven. Table 1 summarizes the number of recommended interventions for credentialing by the various groups that will be summarized in the following discussion. The guidelines for vascular surgeons have evolved with the earlier version published in 1993 being criticized for requiring too few diagnostic and therapeutic angiograms and angioplasty procedures. A revised guideline published in 1999 increases the number of qualifying interventions and establishes parity with other guidelines.

The particular guidelines for each specialty should be benchmarks for physicians and hospitals in determining the appropriateness of individuals in each specialty to safely and effectively perform endovascular procedures. This is particularly important as each specialty's guidelines have been established and will evolve to accommodate new technologies predicated on the background, training, skills,and techniques used by physicians in each specialty. Thus, a particular specialty's guidelines should not be used to determine the appropriateness of application or credentialing for another specialty that has an entirely different perspective regarding training and methods of application. Controversial differences regarding indications and efficacy are issues that should be addressed separately from credentialing criteria, and differences should be resolved by comparative or randomized clinical trials using recommended reporting standards.[9-11] However, parity in the total number of procedures required for credentialing of different specialties in endovascular techniques seems reasonable and appropriate. The following discussion provides an overview of

TABLE 1.
Number of Catheterizations and Interventions

	SCVIR	SCAI	ACC*	AHA*	SVS/ISCVS (1993)*	SVS/ISCVS* (1998)
Catheterizations/angiograms	200	100/50†	100	100	50†	100/50† catheterizations
Interventions	25	50/25†	50/25†	5/25†	10/15†	50/25† procedures
Live demo	Yes	Yes	Yes	Yes	Yes	Yes

*Includes knowedge of thrombolysis or thrombolytic therapy.
†As primary interventionalist.
Abbreviations: SCVIR, Society of Cardiovascular and Interventional Radiology; *SCAI,* Society for Cardiac Angiography and Interventions; *ACC,* American College of Cardiology; *AHA,* American Heart Association; *SVS/ISCVS,* Society for Vascular Surgery/International Society for Cardiovascular Surgery.
(Reprinted with permission of White RA, Hodgson K, Ahn S, et al: Endovascular interventions training and credentialing for vascular surgeons. *J Vasc Surg* 29:177-186, 1999.)

the content of different credentialing documents and outlines areas in which varying recommendations are made for a particular specialty or intervention.

Several articles have been written that address the performance of peripheral endovascular procedures, with most addressing the needs of a particular subspecialty rather than globally addressing the requirements for an endovascular specialist. This has occurred because each subspecialty has dramatically different backgrounds and training requirements to meet the needs of current interventional practice. Interventional cardiologists and radiologists have viewed endovascular surgery from their perspective and training in their individual subspecialties, with expertise in delivery systems and diagnostic modalities that are important in performing current interventional cardiology and radiology procedures. Vascular surgeons have viewed the adaptation of endovascular technologies from the perspective of using catheter-based methods as ancillary techniques to current surgical practice. With the evolution of endovascular technologies the surgical training base has expanded, so that the current focus on endovascular techniques and training is rapidly expanding, with many of the current endoluminal graft protocols for large-vessel devices being heavily dependent on surgical skills in the selection and treatment of patients and for the treatment of complications.

MULTIDISCIPLINE GUIDELINES

One of the most widely referenced publications was in *Circulation* in 1992 by a writing group of the Councils of Cardiovascular Radiology, Cardiothoracic and Vascular Surgery, and Clinical Cardiology of the American Heart Association.[4] This guideline suggests that basic training for peripheral angioplasty include eligibility or certification by the American Board of Radiology, the American Board of Internal Medicine (ABIM) with additional completion of a fellowship in vascular medicine, or the ABIM with additional eligibility of certification in cardiovascular medicine. Eligibility or certification by the American Board of Surgery with additional completion of a general vascular surgery residency was also delineated. Recommended training included previous experience in peripheral angiographic diagnosis and percutaneous transluminal angioplasty, with acceptable complication and success rates. The article notes that the interventionalist should be able to provide documentation of performance of 100 diagnostic angiograms, 50 peripheral percutaneous angioplasties (one half as the primary operator), and 10 peripheral thrombolytic procedures. The report also mentions qualification by apprenticeship, which would be acquired through knowledge of peripheral and visceral vascular disease and angiographic and radiologic equipment and safety. This type of certification would require the same number of procedures as outlined with at least half of the procedures being performed by the interventionalist. The procedures must be performed under direct supervision of a qualified physician preceptor. This proctoring consisting of at least 10 peripheral percutaneous angioplasties. In additon, postgraduate courses including at least 50 category I CME credits in peripheral angioplasty and interventional techniques were suggested. This report is currently outdated with the requirement for the 100 diagnostic angiograms delineated by a specific definition. This definition requires "percutaneous passage of the catheter into an artery under fluoroscopic guidance with subsequent inspection of contrast, material and imaging of the entire vascular distribution in question using conventional serial film changers or large field digital imaging systems. For example, peripheral angiography of the lower extremity vessels must image the vessels of both lower extremities from the distal aorta to at least the ankles." Conventional radiography or video fluoroscopy alone were not considered sufficient for a routine recording of peripheral angiographic studies. Although this criterion fits with a requirement for some interventional radiology programs, current endovascular procedures do not require the strict definition of diagnostic angiography as presented. In many institutions, limited angiographic studies using video fluoroscopy or digital acquisition without fixed film recording is the practice. Experience with the newer methods is more appropriate than the described angiographic technique.

An additional limitation of the American Heart Association guideline is that maintenance of privileges would not be continued for physicians unless they acquire the level of training suggested in the report within 3 years. This requirement is restrictive for individuals who are already successfully practicing endovascular procedures and has no functional basis other than to fulfill a political agenda.

An additional attempt at producing multidisciplinary guidelines was made by the Society for Cardiac Angiography.[3] The suggested guidelines recommend board certification or eligibility in cardiovascular disease or radiology or special certification in vascular surgery or vascular medicine. For cardiology, a cardiovascular training program meeting the requirements of the ABIM and the subspecialty of cardiovascular disease is recommended. For vascular medicine, recommendations include a full training program meeting the requirements of the ABIM plus an additional 2- to 3-year program in the specialty of vascular medicine. Fellowship programs for cardiologists, radiologists, vascular medicine specialists, or vascular surgeons should include extensive experience in general arterial and venous catheterization, in particular, studies referable to the peripheral circulation, including renal and infrapopliteal vessels. The training program should also include a minimum of 12 months of full-time experience in the invasive laboratory and performance of a minimum of 100 diagnostic peripheral angiographic studies (at least half as the primary operator). Additional experience should include 50 peripheral angioplasty procedures (at least half as primary operator) before independent interventions are accomplished. Fifteen peripheral thrombolytic procedures are also recommended.

This report further described that a cardiologist may be able to acquire training during a 3-year fellowship or as an additional year of training. A radiologist could acquire this training during a 1- or 2-year fellowship that follows a standard radiology residency. A vascular surgeon would acquire the training during an extended vascular surgery fellowship. On the basis of this training, temporary privileges would be obtained by providing documentation of procedures performed and identifying those as primary operators, the sites of the lesions treated, the complications, and a letter from the program director. Privileges for physicians not having previous formal training should be obtained by attending at least one live demonstration PTA seminar, learning anatomy indications, and observing at least 10 procedures by an experienced person. The physician would also learn the technical aspects of x-ray usage and the theory of thrombolytic therapy. This training would then be further developed by an apprenticeship with a senior qualified physician who would instruct the candidate in not less than 100 peripheral diagnostic angiographic procedures and 50 peripheral angioplasties (primary operator on at least 50%). The guideline also suggested that the trainee perform at least 15 thrombolytic procedures and that they meet the criteria of the American College of Cardiology/American Heart Association (ACC/AHA) Task Force on PTCA. Once physicians who do not have formal training met these criteria, they would have temporary privileges extended to perform 10 proctored procedures. If no complications occurred, the operator would continue under proctorship until 25 procedures were completed. After 25 cases, with a success rate of at least 85% and a complication rate of less than 5%, the candidate could apply for full privileges. After approval, an annual review by a multidisciplinary panel would review cases and make recommendations to the department chairman or credentialing committee regarding continuation of privileges.

INTERVENTIONAL RADIOLOGY GUIDELINES

The requirements of the Accreditation Council for Graduate Medical Education (ACGME) special training in vascular and interventional radiology include graduation from an approved residency in diagnostic radiology with a minimum of 1 or 2 additional years of training. During this interval, 500 cases including arteriography, venography, angioplasty and related percutaneous revascularization procedures, embolectomy, and percutaneous placement of endovascular prosthesis, stents, and inferior vena cava filters are to be obtained.[12]

The radiology requirements have been further defined in additional publications primarily prepared by the Society for Cardiovascular and Interventional Radiology[2,3,13] and assumes that the physicians have a knowledge of vascular disease and know alternative therapies including risks and benefits. The physician should be competent to interpret diagnostic peripheral and renal angiographic examinations and have further training beyond that necessary for routine diagnostic angiography. This includes being competent to perform angiographic procedures via femoral antegrade or retrograde, axillary, and translumbar approaches.

The minimum requirements are outlined in the radiology requirements of an approved residency program, which includes the criteria described. The performance of the substantial number of peripheral and selected vascular procedures for at least 5 years with acceptable complication rates is recommended. Completion of an approved residency program is optimal and includes instruction in radiation physics, with successful completion of a formal examination on these subjects. Additional experience should include 1 or 2 years postresidency training in percutaneous interventions, which includes participation in a substantial number of peripheral and renal angioplasty procedures, or 200 peripheral and renal angiograms performed within the previous 3 years, with documented success and completion rates within acceptable limits, and participation in a minimum of 25 peripheral and/or renal angioplasty procedures under the direct supervision of individuals who meet these criteria, or the performance of a substantial number of peripheral and renal angioplasties for a period of at least 3 years with documented success and completion rates within an acceptable limit. The radiology documents also include descriptions of facilities that are necessary to perform the procedures. These will not be further discussed in this chapter.

INTERVENTIONAL CARDIOLOGY GUIDELINES

The interventional cardiology community has developed several reports that focus on peripheral angioplasty credentialing and training. An example is the article prepared by the American College of Cardiology Peripheral Vascular Disease Committee published in the *Journal of the American College of Cardiology* (JACC) in 1993.[5] This report suggested that training should include a formal hands-on program in peripheral angioplasty and other vascular interventions acquired by completion of a structured cardiovascular (cardiology) or radiology fellowship, or formal training obtained as part of a vascular surgery residency after board certification in general surgery. An additional acceptable criterion is a vascular medicine fellowship after board certification in internal medicine. Basic understanding of the natural history of atherosclerosis, noninvasive patient assessment, indications, and risks for various procedures are required.

The JACC publication suggested that physician qualifications be documented in formal fellowships that were supported by a letter from the program director. The performance of 100 peripheral diagnostic peripheral angiograms, 50 angioplasties (greater than 50% as the primary operator), and 10 thrombolytic cases was suggested. Postgraduate physicians with or without prior peripheral angiographic experience and without previous angioplasty experience should attend at least two peripheral angioplasty seminars with one live demonstration. The physician should obviously know about atherosclerotic vascular disease, alternative therapies, and noninvasive evaluations. The postgraduate physician should visit peripheral angioplasty laboratories and observe at least 10 cases. He should have angiographic experience with 100 peripheral angiograms, 50 angioplasties (greater than 50% as the primary operator), and 10 thrombolytic cases.

An update of the guidelines for the performance of vascular interventions by cardiologists has been published.[8] The need for this document was supported by advances in the field and by a recent effort by cardiology programs to globally train their fellows to treat peripheral vascular disease. The guidelines outline both limited and unrestricted competency criterion for iliac and renal angioplasty and also outline treatment criteria for peripheral angioplasty.

VASCULAR SURGERY GUIDELINES

The vascular surgery interest in endovascular procedures has increased over the last 15 years related to advances in devices used to treat larger blood vessels. The initial vascular surgery recommendations for quality assurance and development of credentialing were published in 1989,[1] with two subsequent revisions[6,7] further defining the training requirements as the field evolved. The original publications were prepared when vascular surgical participation in percutaneous transluminal angioplasty and stenting of peripheral vessels was limited. Training programs did not address development of catheter-based skills, and the impact of endovascular methods on conventional vascular surgical practice was limited. During the last decade, the development of additional endovascular interventions, in particular endovascular prostheses for the treatment of aneurysms and occlusive disease, has greatly stimulated the involvement and need for surgical expertise. As a result, the vascular surgery training programs have incorporated catheter-based methods as a requirement.

The original vascular surgery training and credentialing guidelines were criticized for not requiring a larger number of interventions to train surgeons to perform angioplasty procedures.[6] The most recent document that was prepared by an ad hoc committee of the Society for Vascular Surgery/International Society for Cardiovascular Surgery has revisited appropriate training methods for vascular surgeons, with the goal being to prepare guidelines that encompass the entire field of endovascular surgery.[7] This encompasses access procedures, positioning of catheters in various locations, and assessing lesions before, during, and after treatment. The range of treatment modalities not only includes balloon dilatation and stenting, but also principles that will be required to select and treat patients with endovascular prostheses. The new document was written to accommodate the rapid evolution that has occurred in the field and is based on current methods used by vascular surgeons to acquire competence. The guidelines have also been written from the perspective that they may not apply to other interventional subspecialties performing endovascular procedures.

The guidelines emphasize that specific skills, such as catheterizations, should be the focus of training rather than less demanding procedures, such as angiograms. The guidelines also recognize that the diversity of vascular surgical practice includes a variety of procedures that fulfill various requirements. For this reason, specific requirements for catheterization and procedures (interventions) were established.

Definition of various types of catheterizations such as direct catheterizations for intravascular introduction and imaging are described. In addition, selected catheterizations were identified as a specific skill and require placement of catheters in branch vessels of a major artery beyond the site of catheter introduction. To provide accounting for catheterizations performed, the highest-order catheterization for a specific vascular branch is counted, not all the vessels that are traversed by the catheter. As an example, bilateral common carotid artery catheterizations from the groin would include one selective aortic catheterization, one first-order left common carotid catheterization, and one second-order right carotid cannulation.

The new vascular surgery training guidelines require senior level participation in at least 100 catheterizations and 50 interventions. The trainee must be primary interventionalist on at least 50% of the procedures, while being no less than first assistant on the remaining 50%. Of the 100 required catheterizations, at least 50% should be selective (first order or greater) and at least 50% should be percutaneous. Of the total number of catheterizations, 75% should be arterial. Of the 50 interventions that are required, 75% should be arterial with less than 25% being venous or dialysis access procedures. In addition, the 100 catheterizations and 50 interventions must be completed during a 2-year interval to ensure a concentrated training experience. Mentors for the fellows or preceptors must have endovascular experience sufficient to meet the training requirement.

The new vascular surgery guidelines have developed a parity in the relative number of required catheterizations and interventions with those suggested by other subspecialties (Table 1). Although an absolute requirement of similar numbers is not thought to be necessary, establishing a minimum that ensures safe and effective performance of procedures is mandatory.

FUTURE PERSPECTIVE

As the endovascular technologies continue to develop and more devices become approved for use, the need to increase the training requirements and the complexity of training has also increased. For the future, all subspecialties need to address the adoption of endovascular methods from the perspective that the interventionalist or the team of interventionalists involved must be able to diagnose, treat, and safely ensure treatment of complications so that patient care is optimized in all scenarios. Multidiscipline efforts to accomplish this goal should be encouraged, with evolution of the ideal vascular interventionalist remaining to be defined.

REFERENCES

1. String ST, Brener BJ, Ehrenfeld WK, et al: Interventional procedures for the treatment of vascular disease: Recommendations regarding quality assurance, development, credentialing criterion, and education. *J Vasc Surg* 9:736-739, 1989.
2. Spies JB, Bakal CW, Burke DR, et al: Guidelines for percutaneous transluminal angioplasty. *Radiology* 177:619-626, 1990.
3. Wexler L, Dorros G, Levin DC, et al: Guidelines for performance of peripheral percutaneous transluminal angioplasty. *Cathet Cardiovasc Diagn* 2:128-129, 1990.
4. Levin DC, Becker GJ, Dorros G, et al: Training standards for physicians performing peripheral angioplasty and other percutaneous peripheral vascular interventions. *Circulation* 86:1348-1350, 1992.
5. Spittell JA, Creager AA, Dorros G, et al: Recommendations for peripheral transluminal angioplasty: Training and facilities. *J Am Coll Cardiol* 21:546-548, 1993.
6. White RA, Fogarty TJ, Baker WM, et al: Endovascular surgery credentialing and training for vascular surgeons. *J Vasc Surg* 17:1095-1102, 1993.
7. White RA, Hodgson K, Ahn S, et al: Endovascular interventions training and credentialing for vascular surgeons. *J Vasc Surg* 29:177-186, 1999.
8. Babb J, Collins TJ, Cowley MJ, et al: Revised guidelines for the performance of peripheral vascular interventions. *Cathet Cardiovasc Interventions* 46:21-23, 1999.
9. Rutherford RB, Flanigan DP, Gupta SK, et al: Suggested standards for reports dealing with lower extremeity ischemia. *J Vasc Surg* 4:80-94, 1986.
10. Ahn S, Rutherford R, Becker G, et al: Reporting standards for endovascular procedures. *J Vasc Surg* 17:1103-1107, 1993.
11. Ahn S, Rutherford R, Johnston KW, et al: Reporting standards for infrarenal endovascular abdominal aortic aneurysm repair. *J Vasc Surg* 25:405-410, 1997.
12. Special requirements for subspecialty training in vascular and interventional radiology. *J Vasc Interv Radiol* 2:303-306, 1991.
13. Waltman AC, Katzen B, Ring E, et al: Society for Cardiovascular and Interventional Radiology: Credentials criterion for peripheral, renal and visceral percutaneous transluminal angioplasty. *Radiology* 167:452, 1988.

CHAPTER 13

Management of Cardiac Comorbidity in Vascular Disease: The Use of β-Blockade

Don Poldermans, MD, PhD, FESC
Consultant, Internal Medicine, Department of Vascular Surgery, Erasmus
Medical Centre, Rotterdam, The Netherlands

Hero van Urk, MD, PhD
Professor Vascular Surgery, Head of Department of Vascular Surgery,
Erasmus Medical Centre, Rotterdam, The Netherlands

Peripheral vascular disease is an increasing problem in Europe and in North America. For example, between 1980 and 1995 in The Netherlands, the number of patients admitted annually to hospitals because of peripheral vascular disease increased from 17,511 to 29,346, an increase of 36% after correction for demographic factors.[1] Although the perioperative cardiac event rate has declined during the past 30 years, the 30-day operative mortality rate for major vascular surgery remains near 6%, and the 5-year mortality rate is about 45%. Cardiac events cause most of this mortality.[2]

The aim of the managing physician is not only that patients should emerge from the operation intact, but also that they should survive long enough to enjoy the benefits of the surgery. Therefore, it is mandatory that the treating physician evaluates the presence and extent of coronary artery disease (CAD) as well as other cardiac risk factors, such as hypertension and hypercholesterolemia, that will determine long-term survival after surgery.

PATHOPHYSIOLOGY OF PERIOPERATIVE CARDIAC COMPLICATIONS

The most clinically significant perioperative cardiac event is myocardial infarction (MI), either fatal or nonfatal. The pathophysiology of perioperative infarction is probably similar to that encountered in the general population. Infarctions occur most frequently on the second or third postoperative day but are not limited to this period.[3] The principal cause of perioperative infarction appears to be fissuring or rupture of a coronary atherosclerotic plaque, with subsequent thrombosis. This phenomenon results from the interaction of neurohumoral factors and hemostatic changes occurring during surgery. Such events occur most often in patients with diffuse, hemodynamically significant CAD. However, some perioperative infarcts may be caused by a sustained imbalance in the myocardial oxygen supply-demand ratio in patients with stable coronary obstructions. Increased myocardial oxygen demand may result from hypertension and tachycardia related to surgical stress, pain, interruption of β-blockers, or the use of sympathomimetic drugs. Decreased supply may be the result of hypotension, vasospasm, anemia, and hypoxia. In contrast to perioperative cardiac events, long-term complications are more common in the presence of left ventricular dysfunction and ischemia.[4]

PERIOPERATIVE CARE

Preoperative evaluation is best done in a stepwise manner. The first step involves taking a careful clinical history and evaluating the risk associated with the planned surgical procedure. Based on the number of clinical risk factors and the proposed surgical procedure, additional tests are planned. Dobutamine stress echocardiography (DSE) and myocardial perfusion imaging are most widely used for the assessment of underlying CAD. Both tests have a comparable specificity for the prediction of perioperative cardiac events, but the sensitivity of stress echocardiography may be superior (Fig 1).[5] However, when stress echocardiography is compared with perfusion scintigraphy, one should consider the limited number of patients studied with stress echocardiography and the more widespread use of perfusion scintigraphy. So far, the use of stress echocardiography has been restricted to a limited number of sites with particular expertise. It remains to be seen whether the results reported from these specialized cardiovascular units can be duplicated in the vascular surgery population at large. The test of choice should be the one with which a given center has the most experience. The presence of inducible myocardial ischemia or reversible

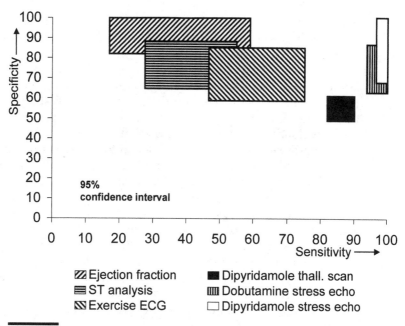

Ⓩ Ejection fraction ▨ Dipyridamole thall. scan
▤ ST analysis ▦ Dobutamine stress echo
▧ Exercise ECG ☐ Dipyridamole stress echo

FIGURE 1.
Meta-analysis of predictive value for perioperative cardiac events in patients undergoing major vascular surgery. (Courtesy of Poldermans D, Bax JJ, Thomson IR, et al: Role of dobutamine stress echocardiography for preoperative cardiac risk assessment: A diagnostic tool comes of age. *Echocardiography* 17:79-94, 2000.)

perfusion defects increases the risk of surgery in proportion to the severity and extent of the induced abnormalities.[5-8]

PERIOPERATIVE β-BLOCKER USE

The optimal treatment for vascular surgery patients with a positive noninvasive test for CAD is still unanswered. Treatment with β-blockers in patients with inducible ischemia and without conventional indications for myocardial revascularization was controversial until recently. In a multicenter randomized study, the cardioprotective effect of β-blockers was clearly demonstrated. The DECREASE (Dutch Echocardiographic Cardiac Risk Evaluation Applying Stress Echo) study evaluated the cardioprotective effect of bisoprolol, a selective β-blocker, in high-risk patients undergoing major vascular surgery.[9] High- risk patients were defined as patients with one or more cardiac risk factors, or a reduced exercise capacity and a DSE positive for myocardial ischemia. These patients were randomly assigned to receive either standard care or standard care plus bisoprolol. During the first 30 days after surgery, the incidence of "hard" cardiac events (ie, cardiac death and MI) was 34% in the control group versus 3.3% in the bisoprolol group ($P < 0.001$). This was the first study showing a cardioprotective effect of β- blockers in a large randomized study population. Mangano et al[10] performed the only previous randomized study evaluating the cardioprotective effect of β-blockers.[10] A total of 200 patients were randomly assigned to receive either atenolol or placebo during the perioperative period. In contrast to the DECREASE study, there was no difference in perioperative mortality, but during a 2-year follow-up, there was a reduction in late mortality in the group of patients given atenolol perioperatively. The apparent lack of a perioperative cardioprotective effect of atenolol in Mangano's study is probably related to the small sample size and the low risk of the study population. Patients were selected by risk factors and not by an objective noninvasive assessment that used either stress echocardiography or nuclear imaging. The low pretest likelihood of cardiac events probably explains the negative results of the study.

The effect of β-blockers on perioperative ischemia was studied by Stone et al.[11] In 128 hypertensive patients, they studied the effect of a small preoperative dose of β-blocker (labetolol, atenolol, or oxprenolol) on the incidence of intraoperative myocardial ischemia. Myocardial ischemia was studied by continuous electrocardiographic monitoring. As expected, the peak heart rate was lower in patients randomly assigned to receive β-blockers (79 vs 100 beats/min [$P < .01$]). Myocardial ischemia occurred in 11 of 39 control patients versus 2 of the 89 patients pretreated with β-blockers ($P < .01$). Wallace et al[12] confirmed the favorable effects of β-blockers on the incidence of perioperative ischemia assessed by continuous electrocardiographic monitoring in 200 patients randomly assigned to either placebo or atenolol. Neither study showed a reduction of perioperative cardiac events. Besides β-blockers, other interventions may reduce perioperative ischemia. For instance, anaesthetic techniques, temperature control, careful monitoring of fluid balance, pain relief, and anticoagulation may reduce perioperative ischemia.

Coronary revascularization in high-risk patients, before major vascular surgery, seems to be an attractive option. However, there are several pitfalls. First, the number of patients with peripheral vascular disease is increasing, and about 10% to 20% of these patients have a positive noninvasive test for CAD. Because surgery is often performed on short notice, this will create a great burden on the revascularization centers. Second, the benefit of "preventive" coronary artery revascularization has not been proven, as discussed in the guidelines for perioperative cardiovascular evaluation for noncardiac surgery.[8] There are only retrospective data about the cardioprotective effect of revascularization in patients undergoing vascular surgery. The Coronary Artery Surgery Study (CASS) registry from 1978 to 1981 contains data on study patients who underwent major noncardiac surgery. The perioperative mortality in patients with CAD who had undergone revascularization was reduced (0.9% vs 2.4%) compared with patients who had not been revascularized.[8,13] However, if the additional mortality rate associated with myocardial revascularization before noncardiac surgery is also considered, the reduction in perioperative mortality associated with revascularization may be minimal. However, long-term survival may be enhanced by myocardial revascularization. An accepted policy is to perform revascularization only in those patients with conventional indications for coronary bypass surgery (eg, those with left main disease or multivessel disease combined with impaired left ventricular function, class III or IV angina unresponsive to medical therapy, or unstable angina).

POSTOPERATIVE β-BLOCKER USE

The optimal approach to improve long-term survival after vascular surgery is unclear. Potential strategies are myocardial revascularization and long-term administration of β-blockers. So far, only perioperative β-blockade has been prospectively demonstrated to reduce the risk of late cardiac events.[10,12] We studied the effect of long-term bisoprolol administration on the incidence of late cardiac events among the surviving high-risk patients from the DECREASE study. A total of 101 survivors were followed up for nearly 2 years after surgery. During follow-up, 21 cardiac events occurred, 7 (12%) in the patients who continued to take bisoprolol and 14 (32%) in the standard care group ($P < .01$). This reduction in cardiac events could not be explained by differences in demographics or a change of medical therapy.

BENEFICIAL EFFECTS OF β-BLOCKERS

β-Blockers are well established in the treatment of ischemic heart disease and heart failure and have shown to improve outcome in nonsurgical patients'.[14] We also showed that perioperative β-blockade with bisoprolol markedly reduces the risk of perioperative MI and cardiac death in high-risk vascular surgery candidates.

Thus, it is not unexpected that prolonged postoperative β-blockade with bisoprolol was also associated with a reduction in the risk of late cardiac death and MI. The mechanisms by which β-blockers exert their protective effect are multifactorial. Proposed beneficial properties of β- blockers include anti-ischemic, antiarrhythmic, and anti–renin-angiotensin effects. In addition, there is an augmentation of atrial and brain natriuretic peptide.[15] There was no increase in the incidence of limb ischemia in patients given bisoprolol. This is further evidence that β-blockade is not contraindicated in the presence of ischemic peripheral vascular disease.

CLINICAL IMPLICATIONS

Several investigations have demonstrated the utility of DSE for preoperative cardiac risk assessment.[5,16-19] Patients with stress-induced new wall motion abnormalities (NWMAs), a hallmark of myocardial ischemia, are at an 8% to 38% risk of cardiac death or MI within 30 days after surgery.[4] In contrast, patients without NWMAs have much lower complication rates: in the range of 0% to 5%. There are, however, significant disadvantages associated with the routine use of DSE (or other noninvasive imaging techniques) in all vascular surgery candidates. These include the substantial costs of the test and, more importantly, the risk of delaying surgery in patients with large aortic aneurysms or critical limb ischemia. The recent DECREASE study demonstrated that perioperative β-adrenergic blockade with bisoprolol reduces the risk of 30-day complications in patients with clinical risk factors and NWMAs to a risk level similar to that observed in patients without NWMAs.[9] This finding raises questions regarding the indications for DSE in patients scheduled for vascular surgery. For example, does simple perioperative administration of β-blockers reduce or eliminate the need for noninvasive preoperative cardiac testing?[20] Is there a subgroup of patients among whom the β-blockers do not effectively reduce the incidence of perioperative cardiac events? Might those patients benefit from myocardial revascularization? To address these issues, we studied the relationship between clinical characteristics, DSE results, β-blocker therapy, and adverse cardiac outcome in a large series of consecutive patients scheduled to undergo major vascular surgery.

In agreement with other studies,[20] analysis of 1351 patients undergoing high-risk noncardiac vascular surgery revealed advanced age, current or prior angina, and a history of cardiac or cerebral ischemic events to be the most important clinical determinants of perioperative cardiac death or nonfatal MI. Apart from clinical data, DSE results were highly predictive of adverse cardiac outcome, which also confirms other investigations.[6] Patients receiving β-blocker therapy had a significantly lower risk than those not receiving such medication; among patients with fewer than three cardiac risk factors, the incidence of perioperative cardiac death and MI was reduced from 2.3% to 0.8%. It should be emphasized in this respect, that patients receiving β-blocker therapy had a considerably worse overall risk profile than those not receiving β-blocker therapy, which makes this result even more convincing. On the basis of a risk score composed of a weighted sum of the prognostic clinical characteristics (age > 70 years, angina, MI, heart failure, diabetes mellitus, stroke, renal dysfunction [serum creatinine level > 180 μmol/L]), a large group (83%) of low-risk patients with fewer than three risk factors could be defined. In this group, the estimated risk of cardiac complications is less than 1%, regardless of DSE results, as long as patients are receiving β-blocker therapy. In the remaining patients with three or more risk factors, those without stress-induced ischemia also had a low estimated cardiac risk in the presence of perioperative β-blocker therapy.

Figure 2 may help to explain how results can be translated into clinical practice. The perioperative cardiac event rate was low (1%) in patients with a clinical risk score of less than 3 points who are receiving β-blocker therapy. Therefore, it seems appropriate to omit DSE (and other noninvasive cardiac testing) in this large (>80%) group of patients and to proceed expeditiously with surgery under protection by β-blocker therapy. DSE is useful to further risk-stratify patients with a clinical risk score of 3 points or more. If protected by perioperative β-blockade, patients without stress-induced ischemia still had a low complication rate (2%) and are also candidates for prompt surgery. Patients with a risk score of 3 points or more and NWMAs (approximately 6% of the population) had a considerable complication rate despite β-blocker therapy. Our data suggest that the proposed treatment policy in these patients may depend on the extent of stress-induced ischemia. Although the numbers of patients and events are relatively small in the specific subgroups, patients with NWMAs in 1 to 4 segments were adequately protected by β-blockers (cardiac event rate, 2.8%). However, in patients with more extensive ischemia (>4 segments), β-blockers failed to reduce the rate of perioperative cardiac complications (cardiac event rate, 36%). Coronary angiography and subsequent myocardial revascularization should be considered in these patients.

The prescription of β-blockers may delay surgery. So far, no study has demonstrated what the optimal run-in period for β- blockers is

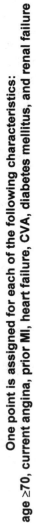

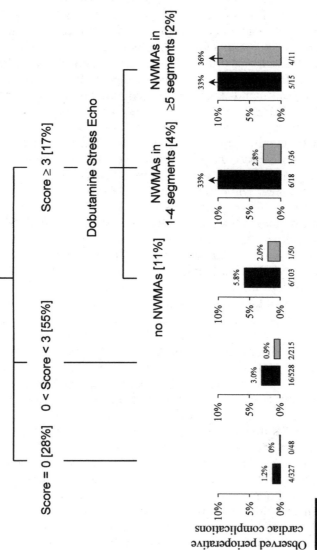

FIGURE 2.

Estimation of perioperative cardiac risk for cardiac death and MI in relation to clinical cardiac risk factors, dobutamine stress echocardiography results, and β-blocker therapy. The *black bars* represent no β-blocker therapy; the *gray bars* represent β-blocker therapy. *Abbreviations: MI,* Myocardial infarction; *CVA,* cerebrovascular accident; *NWMAs,* new wall motion abnormalities. (Courtesy of Boersma E, Poldermans D, Bax JJ, et al: Predictors of cardiac events after major vascular surgery. *JAMA* 285:1865-1873, 2001.)

in this setting. Therefore, it can be questioned whether such therapy is really necessary in patients at very low risk. In the group of patients with a risk score of 0 points, 1.2% perioperative complications were observed in those without β-blocker therapy (Fig 2). This complication rate seems sufficiently low to refrain from therapy and opt for surgery without delay. Another issue is that β-blocker therapy may be contraindicated, especially in patients with reactive airway diseases, such as severe asthma or chronic obstructive pulmonary disease with a reactive component. In the decrease population there were no such cases. Still, if β-blocker therapy is contraindicated, the use of calcium antagonists with a negative chronotropic effect may be considered. The recent INTERCEPT study in post-MI patients reported fewer cardiac events in patients randomly assigned to receive such an agent (diltiazem) as compared with placebo.[21]

CONCLUSIONS

β-Blockers can effectively be used to reduce the incidence of perioperative cardiac events and improve the long-term outcome in patients scheduled for major vascular surgery. In patients with fewer than three cardiac risk factors, additional risk stratification by DSE or other noninvasive testing is unnecessary, provided β-blockers are administered.

REFERENCES

1. Hart- en vaatziekten in Nederland. Dutch Heart Foundation, The Hague, The Netherlands, 1997.
2. Mangano DT: Perioperative cardiac morbidity. *Anesthesiology* 72:153-184, 1990.
3. Dawood MM, Gutpa DK, Southern J, et al: Pathology of fatal perioperative myocardial infarction: Implications regarding pathophysiology and prevention. *Int J Cardiol* 57:37-44, 1996.
4. Poldermans D, Fioretti PM, Forster T, et al: Dobutamine-atropine stress echocardiography for assessment of perioperative and late cardiac risk in patients undergoing major vascular surgery. *Eur J Vasc Surg* 8:286-293, 1994.
5. Poldermans D, Bax JJ, Thomson IR, et al: Role of dobutamine stress echocardiography for preoperative cardiac risk assessment: A diagnostic tool comes of age. *Echocardiography* 17:79-94, 2000.
6. Eagle KA, Coley CM, Newell JB, et al: Combining clinical and thallium data optimizes preoperative assessment of cardiac risk before major vascular surgery. *Ann Intern Med* 110:859-866, 1989.
7. Poldermans D, Arnese M, Fioretti PM, et al: Improved cardiac risk stratification in major vascular surgery with dobutaine-atropine stress echocardiography. *J Am Coll Cardiol* 26:1197-1202, 1995.

8. Eagle LA, Brundage BH, Chaitman BR, et al: ACC/AHA Task Force report. Guidelines for perioperative cardiovascular evaluation for noncardiac surgery. *J Am Coll Cardiol* 27:910-948, 1996.

9. Poldermans D, Boersma E, Bax JJ, et al: The effect of bisoprolol on perioperative mortality and myocardial infarction in high-risk patients undergoing vascular surgery. *N Engl J Med* 341:1789-1794, 1999.

10. Mangano DT, Layug EL, Wallace A, et al: Effect of atenolol on mortality and cardiovascular morbidity after noncardiac surgery. *N Engl J Med* 335:1713-1720, 1996.

11. Stone JG, Foex P, Sear JW, et al: Myocardial ischemia in untreated hypertensive patients: Effect of a single small oral dose of a beta-adrenergic blocking agent. *Anesthesiology* 68:495-500, 1988.

12. Wallace A, Layug B, Tateo I, et al: Prophylactic atenolol reduces postoperative myocardial ischemia. *Anesthesiology* 88:7-17, 1988.

13. Foster ED, Davis KB, Carpenter JA, et al: Risk of noncardiac operation in patients with defined coronary artery disease: The Coronary Artery Surgery Study (CASS) registry experience. *Ann Thorac Surg* 41:42-50, 1986.

14. CIBIS-II Investigators and Committees: The Cardiac Insufficiency Bisoprolol Study II (CIBIS-II): A randomized trial. *Lancet* 359:9-13, 1999.

15. Cruickshank JM: Beta-blockers continue to surprise us. *Eur Heart J* 21:354-364, 2000.

16. Pellikka PA, Roger VL, Oh JK, et al: Safety of performing dobutamine stress echocardiography in patients with abdominal aortic aneurysm ≥4 cm in diameter. *Am J Cardiol* 77:413-416, 1996.

17. Davila-Roman VG, Waggoner AD, Sicard GA, et al: Dobutamine stress echocardiography predicts surgical outcome in patients with an aortic aneurysm and peripheral vascular disease. *J Am Coll Cardiol* 21:957-963, 1993.

18. Lalka SG, Sawada SG, Dalsing MC, et al: Dobutamine stress echocardiography as a predictor of cardiac events associated with aortic surgery. *J Vasc Surg* 15:831-840, 1992.

19. Langan EM, Youkey JR, Franklin DP, et al: Dobutamine stress echocardiography for cardiac risk assessment before aortic surgery. *J Vasc Surg* 18:905-911, 1993.

20. Boersma E, Poldermans D, Bax JJ, et al: Predictors of cardiac events after major vascular surgery. *JAMA* 285:1865-1873, 2001.

21. Boden WE, van Gilst WH, Scheldewaert RG, et al: Diltiazem in acute myocardial infarction treated with thrombolytic agents: A randomized placebo-controlled trial. Incomplete Infarction Trial of European Research Collaborators Evaluating Prognosis post-Thrombolysis (INTERCEPT). *Lancet* 355:1751-1756, 2000.

PART VII

Basic Science

CHAPTER 14

Brachytherapy: Applications for the Vascular Surgeon

David Rosenthal, MD
Clinical Professor of Surgery, Medical College of Georgia, Augusta, Chief of Vascular Surgery, Atlanta Medical Center, Atlanta, Ga

John H. Matsuura, MD
Assistant Professor of Surgery, Medical College of Georgia, Augusta, Atlanta Medical Center, Atlanta, Ga

Vascular brachytherapy for the prevention of arterial restenosis continues to evolve. Recent clinical feasibility reports and early pilot trial data have demonstrated that low doses of radiation after intracoronary transluminal angioplasty reduced neointimal proliferation, prevented vessel contraction, and altered the restenosis rate.[1-4]

Encouraged by early coronary angioplasty results, clinical trials were commenced to evaluate the efficacy of low-dose radiation after femoral popliteal angioplasty and angioplasty of arteriovenous (AV) dialysis grafts.[5-6] A variety of beta and gamma isotopes, and a variety of catheter-based devices, have been advocated for the delivery of low-dose radiation in these peripheral radiation trials. No platform, however, has been developed to deliver low-dose radiation in concert with vascular surgical operations. This chapter focuses on current clinical trial results and current research in the prevention of intimal hyperplasia by brachytherapy for the vascular surgeon.

BACKGROUND

The problem of intimal hyperplasia and hence, arterial restenosis has significant clinical relevance. Information from the Health Care

TABLE 1.
Neointimal Hyperplasia

Operation	No. of Patients
Coronary bypass	250,000
Carotid endarterectomy	150,000
Peripheral bypass	150,000
Dialysis grafts	200,000
TOTAL	750,000
Restenosis rate of 15% =	112,500

Finance Administration demonstrates that in the United States during 1998, approximately 750,000 cardiovascular operations were performed on Medicare-aged patients alone (Table 1).[7] The reported restenosis rates from these operations approaches at a minimum 15% at 2 years, which indicates that more than 100,000 patients may be affected annually by neointimal hyperplasia (NIH). It is obvious that NIH is a major cause of early cardiovascular surgical failures, which results in significant patient morbidity, repeat hospitalizations, and enormous health care costs. Worldwide, these figures may triple.

Vascular injury sets into motion a cascade of events, which may result in the final hyperplastic response of intimal hyperplasia. Stimuli that incite NIH include disruption of the endothelial barrier layer, mechanical factors that disrupt the medial smooth muscle layer, thus serving as stimuli for smooth muscle cell proliferation and migration, and the contact of this disrupted layer with circulating blood factors and mitogens.[8] The principal mechanisms of arterial restenosis are, therefore, acute recoil, intimal hyperplasia as part of the extuberant healing response, and late vascular constriction or "negative remodeling."[9] Vascular remodeling refers to the change in the vascular tone or constriction of the blood vessels. It is an acute process and occurs immediately after percutaneous transluminal angioplasty (PTA). Essentially, when an arterial injury occurs, a race begins between smooth muscle cells traversing the injury site and endothelial cells attempting to repair the injury. Intimal hyperplasia occurs when the smooth muscle cell wins the race.

Radiation therapy has been used for more than 100 years to treat a wide variety of neoplasms by killing the cell or stopping it from replicating. Radiation therapy acts by damaging highly proliferative cells. The growth-inhibiting properties of ionizing radiation

have been used to control benign proliferative disorders, hetero-
topic ossification, keloid formation, ophthalmic pterygia, macular
degeneration, and AV malformations. Compared with the therapeutic doses for cancer treatment (100 Gy), a much lower dose
(1000 cGy) given in a single fraction has been demonstrated to be
effective in controlling the exuberant proliferative response, with
minimal short-term and long-term morbidity. In vitro experiments
showed that low-dose radiation can inhibit the growth of arterial
smooth muscle cells and fibroblasts, and decrease collagen syn-
thesis by fibroblasts. [10] Based on these data and extensive experience with radiotherapy in inhibiting mesenchymal proliferative
processes, it was postulated that radiation may prevent in vivo
intimal hyperplasia in blood vessels and subsequent restenosis.

A simplistic mechanism of action for brachytherapy occurs after
arterial injury and the so-called "activation of humoral defenses"
commences, and a cascade of events is set in motion (Fig 1). The initial stimulus for intimal hyperplasia is the recruitment and activation of immune inflammatory cells (monocytes, macrophages, and T
cells) which are the primary expressors of cytokines and chemo-
kines which are recruited from the circulation and from the vasa
vasorum.[11] At this point, low- dose radiation targets these inflammatory cells in a minimal fashion. The principal effect of radiation,
however, occurs at the point of smooth muscle cell migration and
proliferation where radiation allows the smooth muscle cell to re-

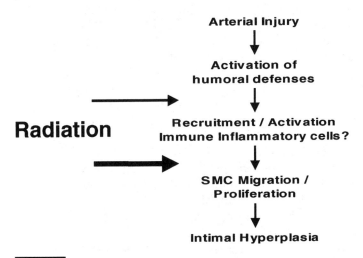

FIGURE 1.
Brachytherapy: mechanism of action. *Abbreviation: SMC,* Smooth muscle cell.

main viable, but unable to migrate or proliferate, thus inhibiting intimal hyperplasia and ultimately arterial restenosis.

Although several low-energy or x-ray–emitting isotopes have been considered for the treatment of NIH, few are currently available at high enough activity to be useful. Gamma isotopes and x-rays deposit relatively little dosage in tissue per radioactive decay, and large amounts of radioactive material (1 Ci or more) are required to yield adequate dose rates. In addition, because of the radiation safety problems associated with gamma x-rays, much effort has been directed towards developing high-energy beta sources. Unlike isotopes or x-rays, beta particles have a finite range in tissue proportional to their energy. Unfortunately, most beta-emitting isotopes with suitable high energy either have a very short half-life or emit significant amounts of gamma radiation as well. Beta emitters used thus far in clinical angioplasty and stent trials are phosphorus 32 (^{32}P), strontium 90 (^{90}Sr), yttrium 90 (^{90}Y), rhenium 188 (^{188}Re), and ^{186}Re. None of these beta isotopes are ideal, either because they have lower energy than desired (^{32}P, ^{186}Re), or too short a half-life (^{90}Y, ^{188}Re), or are difficult to manufacture (^{90}Sr).[12]

BRACHYTHERAPY AFTER PTA IN THE FEMORAL-POPLITEAL VASCULAR SYSTEM

Several radiation systems for peripheral endovascular brachytherapy have been developed,[13] including a high-dose rate after loader, which is a computerized system used to deliver iridium 192 (^{192}Ir) isotope to the treatment site. Radioactive stents with low-activity beta emitters such as ^{32}P are under investigation, whereas another platform to deliver radiation to the peripheral arteries is the use of liquid-filled balloons with isotopes such as ^{188}Re or gas-filled balloons with radioactive xenon 133 (^{133}Xe). These systems offer uniform dose imagery and proximity to the vessel wall; however, special precautions are necessary with these balloon catheters.[13]

FRANKFURT TRIAL

The feasibility of endovascular brachytherapy after PTA in the femoral-popliteal system was first reported by Liermann and recently updated by Schopohl[14] (Table 2). In this 7-year study, 30 patients with in-stent restenosis after femoral-popliteal PTA were treated with stent implant and endovascular brachytherapy of 1200 cGy ^{192}Ir administered by a Micro-Selectron-HDR ^{192}Ir remote after loader (Nucletron Corp, Columbia, Md). The median follow-up was 32.9 months, and the cumulative 5-year patency was 82% based on Doppler ultrasound follow-up.

TABLE 2.
Brachytherapy Trials for Superficial Femoral Artery PTA

Study	Radiation System	Dose (cGy)	Patients	Results
Frankfurt	HDR [192]Ir	1200 at 3 mm	28	Patency at 5 years = 82%
Vienna 02	HDR [192]Ir	1200 at 2.5-3.0 mm	57	Reduced stenosis at 6 months' F/U by 25%
Switzerland	HDR [192]Ir	1400 at 2 mm	Enrolling	In progress
PARIS	HDR [192]Ir	1400 at 2 mm	40	Phase 2 Complete ABI improved

Abbreviations: PTA, Percutaneous transluminal angioplasty; *F/U*, follow-up; *PARIS*, Peripheral Artery Radiation Investigation Study; *ABI*, ankle-brachial index.

VIENNA TRIAL

Pokrajac et al[15] presented preliminary results from an Austrian prospective randomized trial to evaluate endovascular brachytherapy after femoral-popliteal PTA without stent implantation. The mean length of treated arteries was 15.7 cm, and the vessels were treated with 1200 cGy ^{192}Ir delivered by the HDR after loader at a radial distance of 2.5 mm. At 6 months' follow-up in the PTA alone, the restenosis rate was 25%; this was 51.7%, compared with PTA plus brachytherapy arm, which was statistically significant (Table 2).

SWITZERLAND TRIAL

Greiner et al[16] evaluated the effectiveness of brachytherapy in combination with aspirin and probucol, an antioxidant. This 3-tier study will evaluate in phase 1 endovascular brachytherapy with 1400 cGy ^{192}Ir at a radial distance of 3 mm, phase 2 started in parallel with and without endovascular brachytherapy at 5 mm radial distance, and phase 2 will evaluate the effect of aspirin and probucol with and without brachytherapy. Neither centering devices nor stents will be used in this study, and restenosis will be determined as a greater than 50% reduction in luminal diameter by color-flow Doppler ultrasonography.

PARIS TRIAL

The PARIS (Peripheral Artery Radiation Investigation Study)[17] is a multicenter, randomized, double-blind study using a gamma radiation ^{192}Ir source in 300 patients after PTA for superficial femoral

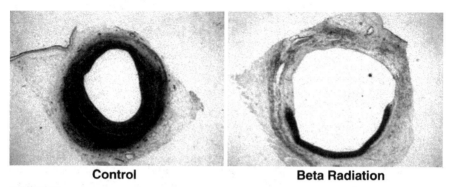

Control   **Beta Radiation**

FIGURE 2.
Brachytherapy-treated aorta.

artery disease. The treatment dose is 14 Gy delivered via a centered segmented balloon catheter using the Micro-Selectron-HDR after loader (Fig 2). In the phase 1 feasibility trial, 40 patients with claudication were enrolled whose lesions had a mean length of 9.9 cm. After PTA and endovascular brachytherapy, the maximum treadmill walking time increased by 1 minute, and the ankle-brachial index (ABI) improved from 0.7 ± 0.2 to 1.0 ± 0.2 (P = .01). The feasibility study of PARIS demonstrated that high-dose gamma radiation delivered via a centering catheter is feasible and safe after PTA for superficial femoral artery lesions.

BRACHYTHERAPY AFTER PTA IN ARTERIOVENOUS DIALYSIS GRAFTS

The most frequently implanted graft in the United States today is the arteriovenous graft (AVG), which has a mean patency of only 15 months because of accelerated NIH formation at the venous anastomotic outflow tract. This aggressive NIH formation is caused by turbulence, compliance mismatch, peritissue vibration, and platelet deposition. Indeed, long-term hemodialysis patients require hospitalization for an average of 1 month each year for placement or revision of their access grafts.[18] Understandably, the vascular access graft has been referred to as the "Achilles heel of the hemodialysis patient."

Parikh and Dattatreyudu[6] reported a trial of fractionated external-beam radiotherapy in 30 patients with AVGs. Fifteen were treated with 8 Gy in two equal fractions 48 hours apart, and the next 15 patients were treated with 12 Gy immediately after PTA of the venous outflow tract. Ten of these patients have follow-up extending to 18 months; all have required "reintervention" to maintain AVG patency, and the study is ongoing.[19] At Columbia Presbyterian Hospital and Duke University Hospital, phase 1 studies evaluating the efficacy of external-beam radiotherapy after AVG placement are ongoing.[19]

BRACHYTHERAPY FOR THE VASCULAR SURGEON

All brachytherapy research thus far has been done with a variety of catheter-based devices and stents. No platform, however, has been developed for the delivery of low-dose radiation in concert with cardiovascular surgical operations. Research has recently commenced using the beta-emitting isotopes tritium and calcium 45 (^{45}Ca) because of their unique characteristics: they both have appropriate half-lives with effective beta energy on contact, yet the radiation exposure to surrounding tissues outside the vessel wall is virtually zero.[20] Indeed, there are essentially no safety issues with the low-dose beta radiation emitted by these isotopes, and the only protection necessary for operating room personnel are latex gloves. No lead aprons, no dose symmetry badges, and no special venting is necessary. Beta radiation has the ability to safely target the vessel wall and not injure surrounding tissues.

It is important to put the amount of radiation exposure used in these studies into perspective. The standard treatment for a head and neck cancer is 70 Gy, whereas the amount of radiation emitted by tritium from a wristwatch (which makes it glow in the dark) is about 20,000 µCi which, if left unshielded, offers a radiation exposure of 1/10,000 Gy. The amount of tritium and ^{45}Ca used on the polypropylene in the studies was approximately 50 µCi. Essentially there is 500 times more radiation exposure from a wristwatch than the labeled polypropylene, which is approximately the same amount of background radiation one gets each day.

In a phase 1 study, the endothelium of rabbit aortas was denuded with embolectomy catheters, and the artery was repaired with 7-0 interrupted polypropylene suture. Ten aortas were repaired with suture labeled with 30 µCi of tritium and 10 with nonlabeled polypropylene suture. Three weeks after operation, the animals were killed and on histopathologic examination of the brachytherapy-treated aortas, there was a significant reduction in medial thickening and hence, increased lumen area (Fig 2). However, there was no consistent evidence of intimal hyperplasia inhibition. Although there was no uniform neointimal inhibition, it was encouraging to note the effects the miniscule dose of beta radiation had on the apparent inhibition of smooth muscle cell replication and migration, a precursor along the pathway for intimal hyperplasia.

Encouraged by these initial results, it was felt that if low-dose beta radiation could be delivered in a more circumferential and linear manner, it would prove to be more efficacious. In a phase 2 study, polypropylene mesh was then labeled with tritium and ^{45}Ca. The endothelium of rabbit carotid arteries was denuded, and the arteries were wrapped with nonradiated mesh (controls), tritium-labeled mesh, and ^{45}Ca–labeled mesh. At 4 weeks' harvest, the denuded surfaces of the vessels were again compared and although there was not a consistent difference between the control and tritium-labeled mesh vessels, between the control and ^{45}Ca–labeled mesh vessels there was a marked reduction in neointimal area, a significant reduction in maximal intimal thickness, and a reduction in percent stenosis, which therefore increased lumen area (Fig 3).

Current trials are underway to identify the most appropriate isotope and dosimetry. An animal trial with AV grafts is planned to determine whether this form of brachytherapy can inhibit NIH at the venous outflow tract of an AV graft. If this simple mesh-wrapping technique inhibits NIH in the animal model, hopefully in the near future we will be able to offer surgical patients this simple and safe means of preventing intimal hyperplasia and, thereby, arterial restenosis.

With any new technology, there is initial enthusiasm, but many questions need to be answered. For example: What are the therapeutic and toxic windows of brachytherapy? What is the ideal dose rate, and will the dose rate be the same for all vessels? Can adjunctive therapy with "radiosensitizers" or other drugs reduce the dose? Are there late radiation effects from even miniscule doses? The cost of arterial restenosis is estimated to exceed $1 bil-

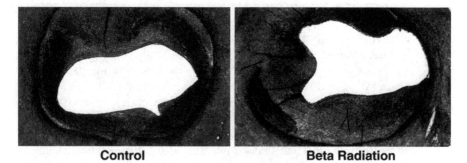

Control   **Beta Radiation**

FIGURE 3.
Control versus brachytherapy-treated denuded rabbit carotid arteries.

lion annually in the United States,[21] and any clinical trials must evaluate the cost-effectiveness of the brachytherapy device. Endovascular brachytherapy for the prevention of restenosis offers our patients a potential adjunctive technology that may dramatically change the practice of vascular surgery.

REFERENCES

1. Carter AJ, Laird JR, Bailey LR, et al: Effects of endovascular radiation from a beta-particle-emitting stent in a porcine coronary restenosis model. A dose-response study. *Circulation* 94:2364-2368, 1996.
2. Laird Jr, Carter AJ, Kufs WM, et al: Inhibition of neointimal proliferation with low-dose irradiation from a beta-particle-emitting stent. *Circulation* 93:529-536, 1996.
3. Waksman R, Robinson KA, Crocker IR, et al: Endovascular low-dose irradiation inhibits neointimal formation after coronary artery balloon injury in swine. A possible role for radiation therapy in restenosis prevention. *Circulation* 91:1533-1539, 1995.
4. King SB, Williams DO, Chougule P, et al: Endovascular beta-radiation to reduce restenosis after coronary balloon angioplasty: Results of the Beta Energy Restenosis Trial (BERT). *Circulation* 97:2025-2030, 1998.
5. Tripuraneni P, Giap H, Jani S: Endovascular brachytherapy for peripheral vascular disease. *Semin Radiat Oncol* 9:190-202, 1999.
6. Parikh S, Dattatreyudu N: Radiation therapy to prevent stenosis of peripheral vascular accesses. *Semin Radiat Oncol* 9:144-154, 1999.
7. *Diagnostic Codes for Short-Stay Hospitals.* Health Care Finance Administration, Office of Information Systems, Medicare Division Support Systems, Office of Strategic Planning, Baltimore, MD, 1998.
8. Schwarte RS: The vessel wall reaction in restenosis. *Semin Interv Cardiol* 2:83-88, 1997.
9. Consigny PM, Bilder GE: Expression and release of smooth muscle cell mitogens in arterial wall after balloon angioplasty. *J Vasc Med Biol* 4:1-8, 1993.
10. Hosoi Y, Yamamoto M, Ono T, et al: Prostacyclin production in cultured endothelial cells is highly sensitive to low doses of ionizing radiation. *Int J Radiat Oncol Biol Phys* 63:631-638, 1993.
11. Rubin P, Williams JP, Finkelstein J, et al: Radiation inhibition versus induction of vascular restenosis, in Waksman R (ed): *Vascular Brachytherapy*, ed 2. Armonk, NY, Futura Publishing, 1999, pp 103-125.
12. Popowski Y: New sources for vascular brachytherapy. Cardiovascular radiation therapy IV syllabus. February 2000.
13. Waksman R: Intracoronary radiation therapy for restenosis: The clinical trials, in Waksman R (ed): *Vascular Brachytherapy*, ed 2. Armonk, NY, Futura Publishing, 1999, pp 435-447.
14. Schopohl B: [192]Ir endovascular brachytherapy for avoidance of intimal hyperplasia after percutaneous transluminal angioplasty and stent

implantation in peripheral vessels: 6 years of experience. *Int J Radiat Oncol Biol Phys* 36:835-840, 1996.

15. Pokrajac B, Potter R, Mac T, et al: Intraarterial ^{192}Ir high-dose brachytherapy for prophylaxis of restenosis after femoropopliteal percutaneous transluminal angioplasty: The prospective randomized Vienna-2-trial radiotherapy parameters and risk factors analysis. *Int J Radiat Oncol Biol Phys* 48:923-931, 2000.

16. Greiner RH, Do DD, Mahler F, et al: Peripheral endovascular radiation for restenosis prevention after percutaneous transluminal angioplasty (PTA). Presented at the Endovascular Brachytherapy Workshop, Napoli, Italy, May 10, 1998.

17. Tripuraneni P, Knowles H, Saeed M, et al: PARIS a multicenter peripheral artery brachytherapy study. Presented at the Endovascular Brachytherapy Workshop, Napoli, Italy, May 10, 1998.

18. Swedberg SH, Brown BG, Sigley R: Intimal fibromuscular hyperplasia at the venous anastomosis of PTFE grafts in hemodialysis patients. *Circulation* 80:1726-1736, 1989.

19. Parikh S: Personal communication, March 2001.

20. Rosenthal D: Prevention of intimal hyperplasia and restenosis: Initial results with a beta energy suture and mesh. Presented at Vascular Endovascular Issues Techniques Horizons, New York, NY, November 16, 2000.

21. Weintraub WS: Evaluating the cost of therapy for restenosis: Considerations for brachytherapy. *Int J Radiat Oncol Biol Phys* 39:949-958, 1996.

Index

S

Information and insights you won't find anywhere else—straight from the experts!

YES! Please start my subscription to the *Advances* checked below with the current volume according to the terms described below.* I understand that I will have 30 days to examine each annual edition.

Please Print:

Name _____

Address _____

City _____ State _____ ZIP _____

Method of Payment

❏ Check (payable to **Mosby**; add the applicable sales tax for your area)

❏ VISA ❏ MasterCard ❏ AmEx ❏ Bill me

Card number _____ Exp. date _____

Signature _____

❏ **Advances in Anesthesia**
$93.00 (Avail. December)

❏ **Advances in Cardiac Surgery**
$97.00 (Avail. January)

❏ **Advances in Dermatology**
$95.00 (Avail. November)

❏ **Advances in Internal Medicine**
$89.00 (Avail. December)

❏ **Advances in Nephrology**
$96.00 (Avail. October)

❏ **Advances in Otolaryngology— Head and Neck Surgery**
$99.00 (Avail. July)

❏ **Advances in Pediatrics**
$89.00 (Avail. July)

❏ **Advances in Surgery**
$85.00 (Avail. October)

❏ **Advances in Vascular Surgery**
$95.00 (Avail. October)

Order your *Advances* today! Simply complete and detach this card and drop it in the mail to receive the latest information in your field.

Your Advances service guarantee:

When you subscribe to an *Advances*, you will receive notice of future annual volumes about two months before publication. To receive the new edition, you need do nothing—we'll send you the new volume as soon as it is available. (Applicable sales tax is added to each shipment.) If you want to discontinue, the advance notice allows you time to notify us of your decision. If you are not completely satisfied, you have 30 days to return any *Advances*.

BUSINESS REPLY MAIL
FIRST-CLASS MAIL   PERMIT NO 7135   ORLANDO FL

POSTAGE WILL BE PAID BY ADDRESSEE

PERIODICALS ORDER FULFILLMENT DEPT
MOSBY
HARCOURT HEALTH SCIENCES
6277 SEA HARBOR DR
ORLANDO FL 32821-9852

VISIT OUR HOME PAGE!
www.mosby.com/periodicals

Mosby
Harcourt Health Sciences

11830 Westline Industrial Drive
St. Louis, MO 63146 U.S.A.